AF598635

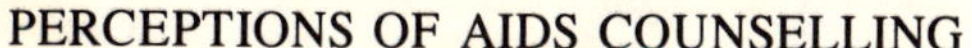

PERCEPTIONS OF AIDS COUNSELLING

Perceptions of AIDS Counselling

A view from health professionals and AIDS counsellors

PHILIP BURNARD
University of Wales College of Medicine

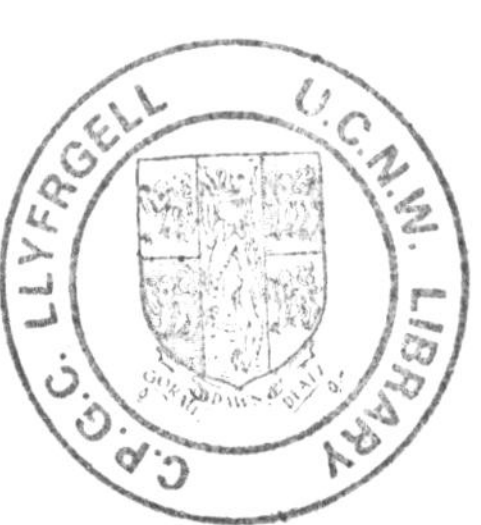

Avebury

Aldershot · Brookfield USA · Hong Kong · Singapore · Sydney

Published by
Avebury
Ashgate Publishing Limited
Gower House
Croft Road
Aldershot
Hants GU11 3HR
England

Ashgate Publishing Company
Old Post Road
Brookfield
Vermont 05036
USA

A CIP catalogue record for this book is available from the British Library and the US Library of Congress

ISBN 1 85628 305 4

Printed and Bound in Great Britain by
Athenaeum Press Ltd., Newcastle upon Tyne.

Contents

About the author

Philip Burnard is Director of Postgraduate Nursing Studies at the University of Wales College of Medicine, Cardiff, Wales, UK and Honourary Lecturer in Nursing at the Hogeschool Midden Nederland, Utrecht, Netherlands. He has also lectured on interpersonal skills and counselling in Brunei, Darussalam and has studied interpersonal skills training in Canada and the USA. He has a Master of Science degree in education from the University of Surrey and a PhD in experiential learning from the University of Wales. He is also a qualified teacher and a general and mental health nurse. He has published 12 textbooks on interpersonal skills, counselling, education, ethics and research methods - including *Counselling Skills for Health Professionals* - and has published numerous journal papers on these and other topics. Dr Burnard's research interests include teaching and learning styles, experiential learning, counselling styles, AIDS counselling and self-disclosure. He is married with two children and lives in Caerphilly, South Wales, UK.

Acknowledgements

Thanks are offered to a number of people who helped in this study. First, thanks to all of the people who gave of their time and agreed to be interviewed. I learned a great deal from them. Particular thanks to my colleague and friend, Paul Morrison, who read parts of the manuscript, made useful suggestions about aspects of the methodology and contributed to chapter two. As ever, thanks to my wife Sally and children, Aaron and Rebecca for their patience and support throughout.

Introduction

Few can be unaware of the urgency of the AIDS issue. Reports continue to tell us that AIDS is still spreading and that hope of a cure is, as yet, some way off. This book offers the findings of a study undertaken to explore AIDS counsellors' and health professionals' perceptions of AIDS counselling - particularly as it relates to nurses and the nursing profession - but also relevant to other health care workers. It was a descriptive study involving the in-depth interviewing of 21 people in the field. Transcripts of the interviewers were produced and subject to four levels of analysis : both quantitative and qualitative. Analysis ranged from one of words, through one of frequently used phrases to more qualitative analyses of the perceptions of the respondents.

At an early stage in the project I became aware that AIDS counselling is a relatively new field. It also differs in some important ways from other sorts of counselling - particularly the more traditional client-centred approach. I found it useful and instructive to continue to make comparisons between AIDS counselling and traditional counselling, throughout the book and these differences are highlighted towards the end of the study. I feel that just as the AIDS situation is changing, so will AIDS counselling. In the early days of AIDS, it seemed as though the accent in counselling was almost exclusively on information giving. Gradually, as the picture has changed, so aspects of AIDS counselling seem to be changing too.

Chapter one offers a review of some of the literature relating to AIDS counselling. Chapter two explores the field of counselling and chapter three identifies and discusses counselling skills. Chapter four reviews aspects of coping with other people's feelings. Chapter five introduces and describes the study and the next two chapters offer the findings of it. The final chapter outlines a model for AIDS counselling training based on the findings and on the literature on the topic. The book closes with a detailed bibliography and an appendix which discusses how the data in this study was analysed with the aid of computer software and an appendix contains the counselling attitude scale used in part of this study.

The study does not claim to be an exhaustive study of AIDS counselling. For one thing, the sheer volume of literature on AIDS and AIDS related issues means that it is impossible for one person to review everything that has been written on the topic. Also, this monograph is something of an interim report. The work reported here is ongoing and research into aspects of AIDS counselling and AIDS counselling in nursing continues. The study does, I trust, raise more questions about the field than it can hope to answer and hopefully adds to the debate about what AIDS counselling may and may not be.

1 AIDS counselling: the background

The number of people being diagnosed as being HIV positive or having AIDS is increasing. There is growing evidence that HIV is spreading in the UK by various means in both heterosexual and homosexual populations (Johnson 1988, Donoghue et al 1989, Pye et al 1989). At the moment, for many nurses, AIDS is a condition that they read about. It is likely, in the future, that many nurses will find themselves caring for people with AIDS (Pratt 1988, Hancock 1991).

Given the unlikelihood of a cure being found for the condition, at least in the short term, it is possible, too, that at a later date, most nurses and health professionals will have personal experience of knowing someone who is HIV positive or who has AIDS (Connor and Kingman 1989; Miller 1990). At present, it seems that AIDS is something that most people have heard of. Fairly quickly, it is becoming something that many people know a little about. The next stage is possibly that each person will know someone with AIDS.

The changing picture

Whilst there are indications that people are beginning to listen to the call for safe sex, there is also evidence that people associate AIDS with being homosexual and that moral positions are still being held

(Wellings and Wadsworth 1990, Fitzpatrick and Milligan 1990). Whilst the notion of AIDS as punishment metered out by God is less popular now, it is still possible to find those who are ignorant about the condition and less than sympathetic to the people who have it (Gaze, 1987; Frankenberg 1990). Wellings and Wadsworth (1990) reporting *British Social Attitudes* noted that 55% of their respondents agreed with the statement that 'AIDS sufferers have only themselves to blame'. It has been suggested that media attempts to change people's attitudes towards AIDS have been less than successful (Kitzinger 1990).

It has also been suggested that AIDS has features in common with epidemics in Europe such as the Black Death of the 14th century (Last 1988). What is less clear is the degree to which such comparisons add to peoples' attitudes towards AIDS and AIDS related conditions. For, as Connor and Kingman (1989) point out :

> AIDS is not, in short, a highly contagious disease, so it is not strictly speaking a 'modern plague', equivalent to the Black Death which decimated Europe in the Middle Ages. (Connor and Kingman 1990 : 3).

These differing viewpoints and perspectives indicate how perceptions of AIDS vary. Given that these opposing viewpoints are offered by experts in the field, it is reasonable to expect that such diversity of perception also exists amongst the general public and amongst nurses.

This chapter considers some of the issues involved in the nurse and other health professionals as AIDS counsellors. It is important to state from the outset that just as not all nurses will need to develop counselling skills in general, nor will all nurses need to develop AIDS counselling skills. It is also important to note that most other health professionals will also need to develop basic counselling skills in this field.

It is possible to argue that the skills involved in counselling the person with AIDS are not fundamentally different to counselling anyone. On the other hand, the evidence suggests that people with AIDS often have particular problems that can best be helped by someone who has specific skills and knowledge (Sketchley 1989, Andersen and MacElveen-Hoen 1988, McCaffrey 1987).

It is notable, too, that nurses and nurse educators are becoming increasingly interested in the issue of counselling as part of the nursing role (Hopper, Jesson and Macleod Clark 1991, Tschudin 1991). Also, it is clear from the developing literature on the topic that AIDS and

AIDS counselling are issues of growing concern to nurses and nurse educators in the UK (see, for example, Hurtig and Fandrick 1990; McGough 1990; Howe 1989; Dennis 1991).

Client groups

Those who receive AIDS counselling are not a homogenous group. A list of the people who are likely to require counselling in this field is offered by Bor et al (1991) :

- Clients who have concerns or queries about AIDS, regardless of their clinical status,
- Clients who are referred for the human immunodeficiency virus (HIV) antibody test,
- Clients who are HIV antibody negative but who continue to present with AIDS-related worries,
- Clients who are HIV antibody positive and symptomless,
- Clients who are HIV antibody positive and who are becoming unwell,
- Clients who have developed AIDS,
- Clients who are being offered, or who are being considered for, antiviral treatments,
- The sexual contacts, loved ones, or family of any of the above, if the client has given his or her permission,
- The close contacts of a deceased client, who may also later require bereavement counselling,
- Staff with concerns about AIDS or those who are occupationally exposed to HIV (in conjunction with the occupational health department) (Bor et al 1991).

Given the diversity of this client group, it seems clear that different sorts of counselling skills and approaches are likely to be needed in AIDS counselling and that 'AIDS counselling' is not one particular entity. Bor and his colleagues (1991) conclude that 'there are many different counselling approaches and no evidence yet that one is better than another.'

For people who are substance abusers, Cook, Fisher, Jones et al (1988) suggests risk reduction counselling which includes :

1. assisting the client to acknowledge the personal risks of HIV infection,
2. explaining the range of changes that will reduce infection and transmission risks, addressing attitudinal and environmental obstacles (for example, feelings of having no control, resistance from partners) and rehearsing behaviours as needed,
3. reinforcing changes in a way that helps the client to assume increasing control over health behaviours so that early accomplishments can be sustained and built upon. (Cook, Fisher, Jones et all 1988).

Faltz (1989) offers the following guidelines for working with substance-abusing clients. Some of these may well be appropriate for other client groups.

- Be willing to listen and encourage constructive expression of feelings,
- Express caring and concern for the individual,
- Hold the individual responsible for his or her actions,
- Ensure consistent consequences for negative behaviours,
- Talk to the individual about specific actions that are disruptive or disturbing,
- Do not compromise your own values or expectations,
- Communication your plan of action to other staff members or professionals working with the client,
- Monitor your own reactions to the client. (Faltz 1989).

A wide range of other sorts of clients have been discussed in the AIDS counselling literature including : 'the worried well' (Bor, Miller, Perry et al 1989), those who want or need to keep their diagnosis secret (Bor, Miller and Salt 1989), the counselling of antenatal women (Miller and Bor 1990), children (Miller, Goldman, Bor et at 1989), those with haemophilia (DiMarzo 1989), and ethnic minorities (Fullilove 1989). Another group that might ask for counselling are bisexual people. The Off Pink Publishing Collective (1988), having noted of the paucity of research into bisexuality write as follows :

> Up until now the fact that maybe over a third of the population has strong attractions to or sexual activities with both sexes has generally been ignored. Sexual self-identities have been seen as either heterosexual, or gay or lesbian. But in reality people are not in distinct groups. As far as disease transmission is concerned, it is actual behaviour rather than self-identify that

counts and many self-identified heterosexuals and gay men and lesbians behave bisexually. Contrary to a frequent association of bisexuality with promiscuity, it is our experience that many self-identified bisexuals are recurrently celibate, and increasingly so as part of a safer sex life.

Reviewing the literature on AIDS, AIDS counselling and sexuality tends to confirm the view that whilst bisexual people are noted to be at risk, they are less widely written about than are gay or heterosexual people.

Some issues for the person with HIV/ AIDS

There are numerous psychosocial issues facing the person who is HIV positive or who has AIDS. Siven and Caldarola (1989) suggest that many gay people who develop AIDS still see themselves as being punished for being gay. This idea can be further fuelled by those without AIDS who continue to suggest that people with AIDS are 'immoral' or 'dirty' (Kitzinger 1990). Also, the person who lives a gay lifestyle and who knows other people with AIDS may well find that they also have to experience the death of friends and may also experience 'survival guilt' if they outlive their friends (Silven and Caldarola 1989).

Friends and families respond and react in various ways to the knowledge that one of them is HIV positive or has AIDS. Not all are supportive and sometimes the person with AIDS has to face rejection by those he or she has loved (Perry and Tross 1984). This may be coupled with the fact of facing AIDS can lead to psychological problems and feelings of dispiritedness and meaninglessness (Silven and Caldarola 1989).

Clearly, there are also a whole range of physical problems to face. The person who is HIV positive may become understandably obsessed with looking for signs of their having AIDS. Once AIDS is diagnosed, the person has to make further adjustments to a wide range of physical and psychological symptoms. Nor need the process be insidious. AIDS dementia, for example, can have a rapid onset and the first signs may be decreasing mental ability, quickly followed by a range of physical symptoms (Boccellari, Dilley and Shore 1988). A discussion of the range and variety of the symptoms of AIDS related conditions is beyond the remit of this chapter but is discussed in detail elsewhere (Miller 1987, Welch and Newbury 1990, Miller 1990).

Much anxiety often surrounds the issue of whether or not to be AIDS tested. The HIV antibody test has been available to those who want to be tested since October 1985 (in the UK). and most Western countries have introduced facilities for such testing. There are specific issues in counselling for the counsellor who faces a person who is unsure about whether or not to be tested. McCreaner identifies the aims of pre-test counselling as follows :

- To ensure that any decision to take the test is fully informed and based on an understanding of the personal, medical, legal and social implications of a positive result. At one level, this is a mere practical application of the traditional medical ethic of informed consent to a procedure,
- To provide the necessary preparation for those who will have to face the trauma of a positive result. Such preparation is vital in that patients who have been prepared for a positive result are able to face that result much more equably,
- To provide the individual, whether he eventually elects not to be tested, or elects to be tested and is found positive or found to be negative, with necessary risk reduction information on the basis of which he can reduce the risk of either acquiring HIV infection or passing it on to others. (McCreaner 1989).

For the person who has AIDS, Sketchley (1989) suggests that there are frequently four stages to be worked through in the counselling relationship :

- Crisis : a stage in which the predominant emotions are shock, fear and denial,
- Adjustment to the news : in which social disruption and withdrawal are common as the person struggles to accept the diagnosis,
- Acceptance : a stage in which the person adopts a new sense of self within the limitations imposed by the illness,
- Preparation for death : a stage in which the issues of fear of dependence, pain, being abandoned, isolation and death, itself, may predominate.

These stages are not at all dissimilar to the stages worked through by any person who has to face the prospect of dying (Stedeford 1989).

The counsellor who seeks to help the person with AIDS may also have to work on his or her feelings about his or her *own* death.

Green offers a comprehensive list of the issues that need to be covered by the AIDS counsellor who is offering post-test counselling and where the result of the test has been positive:

- Breaking the news in a clear and sympathetic way
- Listening carefully to the patient's response and helping him to talk through what it means to him
- Providing facts about HIV and AIDS
- Providing facts about transmission
- Providing information about infection control issues
- Finding out about the patient's sex life
- Finding out about his relationships
- Finding out about any other risk factors. e.g. injecting drug use
- Helping him to implement safer sex
- Helping him to reduce other risk factors
- Helping him to inform sexual partners
- Helping him to deal with relationship issues
- Helping him to arrange a social support network or to make the best use of the one he has
- Informing him about what hospital and voluntary services are available to help him, and how to access them
- Helping him to decide who else he wished to tell
- Encouraging him to take positive steps to maintain and improve general health
- Organising further appointments with the counsellor, and with other health workers,
- Making sure that he has adequate medical support and services
- Helping him with practical problems such as housing, welfare benefits etc,
- Making sure that he knows how to reach the counsellor in case of difficulty and knows he is welcome to seek help from the counsellor. (Green 1989b)

What is noticeable about Green's list is the amount of 'telling' that is involved in AIDS and HIV counselling. Where other sorts of counselling often focus on the drawing out of the client and on the client telling his or her story, the focus in AIDS counselling is often on ensuring that the client has information that can help prevent the spread of AIDS and which can make the quality of the life of the client greater. The question remains, however, whether or not enough emphasis is placed on the emotional and personal aspects of the experience of AIDS. As we will see, other forms of counselling usually place the feelings of the client at the centre of the relationship.

AIDS counselling

AIDS counselling is carried out by many people. At one level, various telephone counselling services exist for people who are worried that they may have AIDS and for those who need support. At another level, there are people who are identified specifically as AIDS counsellors (Leukefeld 1988). They are often attached to hospitals, hospices and national AIDS organisations and offer help to people with AIDS, their friends and families (Dilley, Pies and Helquist 1989).

It is notable that different cities have organised their counselling and support systems in different ways. In 1987, the Canadian Federal Centre for AIDS, observed that the AIDS programme in San Francisco was much more community oriented (with correspondingly more counselling agencies) than was the programme in New York (where many more people were being cared for in hospital).

Increasingly, nurses will find themselves fulfilling the role of AIDS counsellor, for as Bor (1991) points out, they are at the forefront of professional care-giving to patients and families affected with or affected by AIDS. If AIDS continues to increase in incidence (and there is every evidence that it will), then nurses will find themselves caring for more and more people who have developed a range of infections suffered by people with AIDS. At least two things follow from this. All nurses will have to have a considerable knowledge about the nature of AIDS. They will also have to explore their own values and attitudes to the problem and to develop counselling strategies and skills.

On the first issue, the question of nurses developing their knowledge base, the problem is a difficult one. Just as the AIDS virus, itself, seems to be changing (Connor and Kingman 1990), so does the research and knowledge base. No worker in the field can expect to stay completely up to date. On the other hand, certain issues stay the same. The mode of transmission of the virus is well documented and everyone should have a clear idea about what constitutes safe sex and what to do to avoid becoming a person with AIDS (Miller 1987, Miller 1990).

Sketchley (1989) suggests that counselling people with AIDS involves three domains :

- Educational issues.
- Advice.
- Psychosocial issues.

Nurses' attitudes towards and knowledge of AIDS

Nurses' knowledge and views of AIDS and of people with AIDS varies considerably. In an American study by Eakes and Lewis (1991), a total of 40 baccalaureate nursing students were asked to write a paper that expressed their opinions about providing care to patients with AIDS and to give the rationale used to support their views. Although 75% of the students believed that nurses should provide care to patients with AIDS, 25% expressed either negative or ambivalent feelings about providing such care. Moreover, many of the same rationales were offered to substantiate all three attitudes, emphasizing the need for definitive guidelines for decision making.

Klonoff and Ewers (1990) administered a questionnaire to the nursing staff of a large teaching hospital in the USA to determine: 1) sources of stress in caring for AIDS patients; 2) perceived sources of stress in being an AIDS patient; and 3) attitudes towards "deserving" various illnesses. Principal components analyses revealed a number of factors related to increased stress, including: general concerns about the care of these patients; specific concerns in crises situations; and concerns regarding the personal/social implications of caring for these individuals. These factors were not related to either prior experience of taking care of AIDS patients, or nursing specialty. People with AIDS were viewed as "deserving" their illness in much the same way as noncompliant diabetic or renal patients.

D'Augelli (1989) undertook a study of the attitudes and concerns about AIDS of 144 nursing personnel attending conferences on AIDS in rural central Pennsylvania. Participants were knowledgeable about AIDS but wanted to know more and wanted additional training. Most were moderately worried about contracting AIDS, and a sizeable percentage showed irrational fears. AIDS fears cantered around fear of casual-contact transmission and transmission through intimate contact. Participants held generally negative views of gay men and lesbians, and few had personal knowledge of gay people. Homophobic attitudes correlated significantly with AIDS phobias, suggesting that feelings about gay men may influence the nature of medical care that AIDS patients who are gay might receive.

In a study by Goldenberg and Laschinger (1991) forty-six second-year baccalaureate nursing students completed a questionnaire developed according to guidelines described by Ajzen and Fishbein prior to and following a teaching unit on caring for AIDS patients. Students' attitudes and subjective norms were found to be significant predictors of intentions to care for AIDS patients in their clinical experience . In addition, qualitative data resembled those in previous reports of fear of contagion among health professionals. The effects of the teaching unit about caring for AIDS patients resulted in significant changes in both attitudes and subjective norms.

In New Zealand, Wills (1990) carried out a small survey to examine nurses attitudes to a wide range of matters relating to the management of patients and persons with AIDS, and the prevention of HIV infection. Strong support was shown for the current AIDS related public health measures, particularly in the area of health education. Unnecessary measures like mandatory screening have scant support, and there is even less support for more extreme measures. Most nurses believed AIDS patients should be treated no differently than other disease sufferers. While there was an awareness and concern about occupational transmission, most nurses approached or would approach caring for AIDS patients no differently than approaching other patients.

Nurse's needs for AIDS information has also been investigated. A study by Flaskerud (1989) identified 1) the needs of psychiatric nurses for information on AIDS; 2) the groups to whom they provide AIDS education, counselling, and referrals; and 3) their preferred resources for AIDS information. A national survey of 233 American psychiatric nurses was conducted. The most important areas of need for AIDS information were psychosocial aspects of the care of AIDS patients, families, and health care workers; the assessment of AIDS symptoms; and management of psychiatric complications. The nurses provided education and counselling to a wide variety of transmission groups, community groups, and health care workers. They preferred continuing education conferences, journals, and popular print and visual media as resources for AIDS information.

Brown, Calder and Rae (1990) undertook a study to determine if increased knowledge changes nursing students' attitudes toward individuals with AIDS. A pretest/post-test design was used to administer a questionnaire, developed and validated in the United States, and adapted for use in the study. Subjects were total populations of first to fourth year baccalaureate undergraduate nursing students attending a 1-day AIDS workshop. Questions dealt with knowledge and fears concerning AIDS and caring for AIDS patients, and attitudes toward homosexuality and toward the terminally ill. Post-test results indicated that all groups of students displayed a knowledge gain and a more positive attitude toward caring for AIDS patients, particularly by first and third year students. Although positive, younger students and students who had cared for AIDS patients were less positive. In this study, AIDS education had a positive influence on attitudes of nursing students. The researchers suggest that the finding supports the use of education to foster positive attitudes toward AIDS and individuals with AIDS.

Swanson, Chenitz, Zalar, and Stoll (1990) undertook a review of the literature to nurses' knowledge, attitudes, and practices (KAP) concerning acquired immunodeficiency syndrome (AIDS) and human immunodeficiency virus (HIV) infection, and care of people with AIDs (PWAs). Areas reviewed included the following: (1) KAP studies of health professionals that include nurses; (2) KAP studies of nurses; (3) KAP studies of nursing students and faculty; (4) studies of stress and coping related to care of PWAs; and (5) studies of outcomes of AIDS education programs. Gaps in knowledge and negative, fearful attitudes toward HIV transmission and PWAs were identified. Negative fears and behaviours decreased in nurses with the gain in accurate information. The studies were largely atheoretical descriptive surveys of health professionals in acute care settings. The authors conclude that studies of nurses specifically, including more studies of obstetric and paediatric nurses, and nurses in a range of settings in the community would be beneficial both in the United States and in other countries.

It would appear from these studies that whilst nurses are possibly a little more knowledgeable of AIDS than the person in the street, they still require considerably more training in the field. It would also appear that they need help in exploring their attitudes towards AIDS and towards people with AIDS. On the other hand, knowledge and attitudes of some other health care workers are little or no better informed. In a study by Knox, Dow and Cotton (1989), mental health care providers completed a set of measures assessing their attitudes, knowledge, and beliefs concerning AIDS. Those surveyed were aware of the main transmission routes but were excessively concerned about casual contact. Most indicated that they are not competent to deal with

AIDS patients and would prefer not to care for them. The majority favoured client testing and segregated programs for HIV-infected persons. Additional AIDS-related education and staff support are needed to overcome irrational beliefs and prejudice.

Gauch, Feeney and Brown (1990) studied the attitudes toward AIDS in 212 people attended an annual meeting of the New Jersey Society for Medical Technology. Twenty five percent of the respondents were considering leaving the profession because of a fear of AIDS. In addition, almost half would not have chosen the field knowing they would be handling HIV-positive samples.

Nurses and AIDS counselling

Bor et al (1991) have offered a useful 'counselling survival kit' for nurses. They suggests ways in which nurses can develop skills in listening and acknowledging the problems and anxieties of people with AIDS in an empathic and accepting way. They also suggest that such nurses must be correctly informed about the nature of AIDS. If Sketchley (1989) is right, nurses will also have to develop their counselling skills in further directions. Under the headings of education, advice and psychosocial issues come a number of sub-headings.

On the issue of education, nurses will be responsible, increasingly for answering people's questions about the AIDS virus and about the likelihood of becoming a person with AIDS. This sort of counselling will be applicable as much to the 'worried well' as to those in high risk groups (Bor, Miller, Perry et al 1989). They will need to know about the modes of transmission of the virus and about its spread. They will also have to become acutely aware of the *vocabulary* in the field. It is reasonable, for example, not to take for granted that people 'suffer' from AIDS. Nor do people necessarily want to known as 'victims'. The idea of being careful about language in this way is not particular new (Giglioli 1982) but has never before been so important to people's self-esteem and morale.

The question of advice will range through a wide variety of variables. On the one hand, those who are HIV positive or who have AIDS will want to know how to seek symptomatic treatment for some of the physical problems they may encounter. They may also still require information about safe sex (Barrick 1989, Roffman et al 1990). As Bor (1991) points out, we should not assume anything about clients' concerns, nor that they have knowledge of AIDS. Having AIDS is no automatic indicator of a person's knowledge about it (Lovejoy and Moran 1988). Nor can it be assumed that information and advice, alone will change people's behaviour. Many other conditions have to be satisfied before knowledge leads to behaviour change (Aggelton 1989; Nelkin 1987). The nurse-as-counsellor will have to be prepared to discuss life-styles and ways of communicating, alongside the giving of advice.

Allied to this question of advice and information is the need to cope with what has been called 'AIDS anxiety' (Folstein 1984). Some homosexual and bisexual people have become increasingly nervous of the prospect of developing AIDS to the point that they develop a number of symptoms of anxiety.

Perhaps prior to working with an advice-giving approach, is an exploration, by the nurse, of her own attitudes towards AIDS and towards people with AIDS. It seems unlikely that the nurse will be all that effective if she or he is disturbed by the prospect of counselling a person with AIDS. Linked to this is the fact that many people find the question of talking about 'delicate issues' difficult (Silverman and Perakyla 1990). This is true of both nurses and their clients.

Also, there is the fact that counselling the person with AIDS may call for a different approach to other sorts of counselling. Many writers on counselling have advocated a 'client-centred' approach (Rogers 1967, Murgatroyd 1985). Essentially, this style of counselling suggests that the starting and finishing point of counselling lies with the client's perceptions and the client's views of their problems. In client centred counselling, the lead is taken by the client and the counsellor remains more and more in the background. The approach can be traced back to the work of humanistic psychologist and father of the client-centred approach, Carl Rogers (Rogers 1951, 1967).

Given the fact that AIDS counselling may involve educating and advising, it is suggested that a more confronting and prescriptive mode may often have to be engaged in. On the other hand, there will also be times - especially in the domains of feelings and emotions - that the counsellor *will* adopt the client-centred approach. Heron (1989) has suggested that counselling can be both 'facilitative' and 'authoritative'. He has indicated that therapeutic interventions can range through six categories : informative, prescriptive, confronting, cathartic, catalytic and supportive. These categories and the implications of their use in AIDS counselling is discussed again later in this book.

In research using Heron's categories, Burnard and Morrison (1988) found that groups of nurses identified themselves as being more proficient in being informative, prescriptive and supportive than they did in being cathartic, catalytic or confronting. Perhaps nurses will have to broaden their interpersonal style when developing their skills in the field of AIDS counselling. Burnard (1989a, 1989b) has described ways that this may be achieved through experiential learning activities.

On the issue of psychosocial problems in AIDS counselling, these seem many and varied. First and foremost would seem to be the person's *own* perception of themselves as a person with AIDS. It cannot be assumed that people with AIDS form an homogenous group who respond to the knowledge of having AIDS in similar ways. Also, there are many different reactions to having AIDS from people from different cultural backgrounds (Fullilove 1989, Sue and Zane 1987). People bring to the experience of having AIDS a wide range of previous life experiences, prejudices, fears, anxieties and attitudes. Some of these may be linked to knowledge levels about the situation. Others, as we have seen, may be linked to societal attitudes and beliefs.

Once individual responses to AIDS have been explored, the question of relationships and other people's responses, occurs. Again, we cannot assume that other people will respond to the knowledge that someone they know and/or love has AIDS in a particular way. Other people's responses are as idiosyncratic as are the ways that the *individual* responds.

After initial counselling about feelings and reactions, come deeper issues about meaning, purpose and dying (Warner-Robbins and Christiana 1989, Marshall and Nieckarz 1988). Such discussions may well take place in the context of deteriorating health which, in turn, may make the task more difficult. The handling of such counselling sessions is likely to call into question the nurses own feelings and their own reactions to the 'ultimate' questions of life (Burnard 1987).

AIDS counselling for nurses

Many courses in AIDS counselling are already available to both nurses and other carers. The question remains, however, to what degree all nurses should undergo some basic training in the field. At the moment, perhaps, it is for individual nurses to identify their own needs and wants. It is questionable how long this state of affairs can be allowed to continue. If, as is suspected, the incidence of AIDS continues to grow, the AIDS issue is going to be everyone's business. In the mean time, more research needs to be undertaken to establish exactly how best to train nurses in helping those with AIDS.

From a review of the literature, three elements of training appear to be important :

- Information about AIDS,
- Values clarification,
- Counselling skills.

It would appear that any training programme for nurses would need to include these elements. First, nurses need up to date and accurate information about the prevention, incidence, nature and characteristics of AIDS and HIV. They also need information about the psychosocial issues involved in being a person with AIDS.

Values clarification is an approach to helping people to explore their beliefs, values and attitudes (Kirschenbaum 1978). Again, it would seem vital that these are examined with nurses prior to those nurses working in the capacity of AIDS counsellors.

Finally, given that the focus of the role is counselling, a grounding in basic counselling skills is essential to any programme of this sort. The skills of questioning, reflecting, empathy building and checking for understanding can be augmented by skills in confrontation and effective information giving (Nelson-Jones 1982, Heron 1986). Whilst, as we have noted, the counselling approach in AIDS counselling may not always be of the client-centred approach, client-centred skills can serve as the basis of a broader range of effective counselling skills.

This chapter has discussed some of the issues involved in considering the training of nurses as AIDS counsellors as part of their nursing role. It has been identified that not all nurses will want or need to take part in such work but that those who do will need to explore their own attitudes, develop a broad and accurate knowledge base and develop a range of effective interpersonal and helping skills.

2 Aspects of counselling

Counselling is widely used as a strategy in health care (Tschudin 1990, Burnard 1989, Bolger 1982, Davis and Fallowfield 1991). This chapter explores some of the issues involved in the process of counselling. On the one hand there is the formal counselling that is offered by counselling agencies such as RELATE (The Marriage Guidance Council). On the other, there is informal counselling that takes place either between friends or colleagues. There is also a more 'medical' aspect to counselling. Davis and Fallowfield (1991) identify, amongst other sorts, the following types of counselling in a health care context:

- counselling in general practice,
- counselling and disfigurement,
- counselling in head injury,
- counselling people with multiple sclerosis,
- infertility counselling,
- genetic counselling,
- counselling families of children with disabilities,
- counselling patients with cancer (Davis and Fallowfield 1991).

As we shall see, AIDS counselling, whilst it has some very particular characteristics, also shares many family resemblances with other forms of counselling. The person who is stressed may choose the anonymity and confidentiality of the professional counsellors or may feel more at home with friends. In that sense, counselling may also be further subdivided : into 'informal' counselling and 'professional' counselling.

Counselling has its roots in a number of traditions, philosophies and psychologies. Woolfe, Dryden and Charles-Edwards (1989) identify a number of key influences, as follows:

- Sigmund Freud and psychoanalysis,
- The Californian personal growth and humanistic psychology movement of the 1950s and 1960s, of whom Carl Rogers has had the most influence on counselling practice,
- More orthodox schools of mainstream psychology out of which have developed a variety of behavioural and cognitive therapies.

Of these three key influences, perhaps the most pervasive has been that of the work of Carl Rogers, within the field of humanistic psychology in general. Rogers is usually thought of as the father of the 'client-centred' approach to counselling which grew out of his early disenchantment with the more prescriptive psychotherapies of the 1940s (Kirschenbaum 1978). The school of humanistic psychology was also the medium through which the individualism of the client-centred approach flourished.

Humanistic psychology

Humanistic psychology was an important influence on the development of counselling and therapy. It developed in the 1940's, 50's and 60's as a reaction to the 'mechanism' of behavioural psychology and the determinism of psychodynamic psychology. Humanistic psychologists argued that people were free to choose their own lives and thus were 'authors' of their own existence. This philosophical perspective drew heavily on the existentialism of Sartre (1955), Heidegger (1927) and others.

Humanistic psychology's main leaders, particularly in the 1960's (which offered exactly the right climate in which humanistic psychology could flourish) were Carl Rogers (1967, 1972, 1952) and Abraham Maslow (1972) [who is said to have named humanistic psychology (Grossman 1985)]. Rogers is particularly well known for his client-centred counselling and for his student-centred learning methods (Rogers 1983). In the 1960's he also developed the encounter group approach to developing self awareness. As we have noted, many of the experiential learning methods described here developed out of the school of humanistic psychology, which, rather like Deweyian educational practices, emphasised the uniqueness of human experience and human interpretation of the world. Rogers had been considerably influenced by Dewey as he had been taught at university by a student of Dewey's, William Kilpatrick (Kirschenbaum 1979).

The 'Articles of Association' formulated by the American Association of Humanistic Psychology at its inception in 1962 described the field in this way :

> Humanistic psychology is primarily an orientation towards the whole of psychology rather than a distinct area or school. It stands for the respect and the worth of persons, respect of differences or approach, open-mindedness as to acceptable methods, and interest in exploration of new aspects of human behaviour.As a 'third' force in contemporary psychology, it is concerned with *topics that have little place in existing theories and systems : love, creativity, self, growth, organism, basic need-gratification, higher values, being, becoming, play, humour, affection, naturalness, warmth, ego-transcendence, objectivity, autonomy, responsibility, meaning, fair play, transcendental experience, peak experience, courage* and related concepts [emphasis added]. (A.A.H.P. 1962 : 2)

These were extravagant claims. Many of the 'topics that have had little place in existing theories and systems' had received the attention of psychologists prior to the formation of the association (presumably, too, concepts such as 'being', 'objectivity' and 'autonomy' had been discussed by philosophers for centuries). By way of example, in psychology, Adler (1927), Horney (1937) and Fromm (1957) had discussed love from the point of view of psychodynamic theory. Creativity had been fairly thoroughly explored by other psychologists (Getzels and Jackson 1962, Anderson 1959). Jung had used the term 'self-actualization' prior to its use in humanistic psychology (Jung 1931) and William James had examined 'peak experiences' and transcendental states in a thorough work at the turn of the century (James 1902).

The tone of the much of the writing in humanistic psychology is American. Yalom, writing in the late 70's, notes that :

> An importation and an Americanization of existential thought and therapeutic procedure has occurred. The frame is European but the accent is unmistakably New World-ish. The Europeans focus is on the tragic dimensions of existence, on limits on facing and taking into oneself the anxiety or uncertainty and non-being. The humanistic psychologists speak less of limits and contingency than of development of potential, less of acceptance than of awareness, less of anxiety than of peak experience... (Yalom 1977).

Other critics were rather more direct when discussing humanistic psychology's approach. Clare described the humanistic psychology movement as part of the 'me generation' culture (Clare 1981). Masson (1990) suggested that Carl Rogers was responsible for producing therapists who were 'the bland showing the not-so-bland how to be bland' and accused Rogers of being politically naive.

It has been argued that there are at least two types of humanistic psychology (Rowan 1989, Mahrer 1989). One is the sort that has a particularly positive view of human beings. People are viewed as having a tendency to 'grow' and develop. At its most extreme, this approach argues that people are essentially 'good' : an idea that dates back at least to Rousseau. It is an idea that has tended to be a reaction against the Protestant and Freudian idea of people as essentially 'evil' or bad (Murphy and Kovach 1972). This 'positive' view of humanistic psychology is typified by writers such as Carl Rogers (1952, 1967) and Abraham Maslow (1972).

The second type of humanistic psychology draws more particularly from existentialism and sees people as neither good nor bad. People, in this version, are completely free. That freedom does not necessarily lead them towards goodness or badness. Essentially, people are 'neutral'. Representative writers of this approach include Rollo May (1989) and Erich Fromm (1957, 1979).

Both types of humanistic psychology acknowledge that people are complex and ever changing. No one theory of how people 'work' would necessarily explain this person in this situation. Humanistic psychology places great importance on how the individual interprets her world and does not seek to develop a 'grand theory' of how human beings think, feel and act. Thus it differs from behaviourism and psychoanalysis which both offer overall explanatory theories of the person.

Client-centred counselling

The term 'client-centred', first used by Carl Rogers (1951) refers to the notion that it is the client, himself, who is best able to decide how to find the solutions to their problems in living. 'Client-centred', in this sense may be contrasted with the idea of 'counsellor-centred' or 'professional-centred', both of which may suggest that someone other than the client is the 'expert'. Whilst this may be true when applied to certain concrete 'factual' problems : housing, surgery, legal problems and so forth, it is difficult to see how it can apply to personal life issues. In such cases, it is the client who identifies the problem and the client who, given time and space, can find their way through the problem to the solution.

The client centred approach was a reaction to the determinism of Freudian psychology (Hall 1954) and the mechanistic approach of the behaviourists. Drawing from phenomenology and from existential philosophy, the client-centred method of counselling put personal responsibility and freedom of choice at the centre of the counselling process. (Dryden, Charles-Edwards and Woolfe 1990). The approach was typical of the therapies generated by the school of humanistic psychology which prospered, particularly, in the 1960's when the zeitgeist encouraged free thinking and liberalism. Rogers' particular approach to client-centred counselling was carried over, by him, into the field of education where he developed the theme of student-centred learning (Rogers 1983).

Murgatroyd (1985) summarises the client-centred position as follows:

- a person in need has come to you for help,
- in order to be helped they need to know that you have understood how they think and feel,
- they also need to know that, whatever your own feelings about who or what they are or about what they have or have not done, you accept them as they are
- you accept their right to decide their own lives for themselves
- in the light of this knowledge about your acceptance and understanding of them they will begin to open themselves to the possibility of change and development
- but if they feel that their association with you is conditional upon them changing, they may feel pressurised and reject your help.

The first issues identified by Murgatroyd, the fact of the client coming for help and needing to be understood and accepted, have been discussed in previous chapters. What we need to consider now are ways of helping the person to express themselves, to open themselves and thus to begin to change. It is worth noting, too, the almost paradoxical nature of Murgatroyd's last point : that if the client feels that their association with you is conditional upon them changing, they may reject your help. Thus we enter into the counselling relationship without even being desirous of the other person changing.

In a sense, this is an impossible state of affairs. If we did not hope for change, we presumably would not enter into the task of counselling in the first place! On another level, however, the point is a very important one. People change at their own rate and in their won time. The process cannot be rushed and we cannot will another person to change. Nor can we expect them to change to become more the sort of person that we would like them to be. We must meet them on their own terms and observe change as they wish and will it to be (or not, as the case may be). This sort of counselling, then, is a very altruistic sort. It demands of us that we make no demands of others.

Client-centred counselling is a process rather than a particular set of skills. It evolves through the relationship that the counsellor has with the client and vice versa. In a sense, it is a period of growth for both parties, for both learns from the other. It also involves the exercise of restraint. The counsellor must restrain herself from offering advice and from the temptation to 'put the client's life right for him. The outcome of such counselling cannot be predicted nor can concrete goals be set (unless they are devised by the client, at their request). In essence, client-centred counselling involves an act of faith : a belief in the other person's ability to find solutions through the process of therapeutic conversation and through the act of being engaged in a close relationship with another human being. Alongside the strategies involved in client-centred counselling go a set of personal qualities that were deemed, by Rogers, to be essential for the carrying out of the approach.

Nurses' attitudes towards client-centred counselling

In a recent study (Burnard and Morrison 1991), a total of 142 nurses were asked to complete and score the Nelson-Jones and Patterson Counselling Attitude Scale (Nelson-Jones and Patterson 1975; see appendix 2). The distribution of that sample is illustrated in Figure 2.1. The sample was a opportunistic one (Field and Morse 1985) in that respondents were taking part in counselling skills workshops run by one of the authors (PB). The instrument was administered at the beginning of the workshop and before any discussion of counselling or counselling skills had taken place.

District Nursing Students	24
Health Visiting Students	24
Staff Nurses (General Nursing)	22
Professional Nurses *	20
Community Psychiatric Nursing Students	21
Qualified Community Psychiatric Nurses	12
State Enrolled Nurses	10
Practice Nurses	9
TOTAL	142

Figure 2.1 : Distribution of the Sample (n=142)

* *The nurses in this group comprised those who were over 30 years of age, with more than 4 years experience of nursing in a position of responsibility. This group was made up of nurse tutors, nurse managers and senior clinical nurses.*

There are a number of clear advantages and disadvantages to this sampling procedure. On the one hand, the opportunistic sample allows for the speedy collection of data from a range of different sorts of people. The method is economical of time, allows easy access and a good response rate. On the other hand, such a sample can never be representative of any total sample and the researcher must be cautious about extrapolating or generalising from his findings. Another issue is that all of the people in this opportunistic sample were participants in counselling skills workshops and therefore it may be reasonably assumed that they were interested in the idea of counselling in nursing prior to completing the questionnaire.

The research instrument

The Nelson-Jones and Patterson Counsellor Attitude scale is a 70 item questionnaire. Respondents are asked to read each item and to respond by indicating that they agreed with, disagreed with or could not decide about each item. Examples of statements from the questionnaire are as follows:

> The counsellor should ask questions only when he does not understand what the client has said.
>
> If a client wants to discontinue counselling, he should be allowed to do so.
>
> The more information the counsellor has about the client prior to the counselling interview, the better he will be able to understand the client.

The scale was devised by Nelson-Jones and Patterson out of work on other scales which attempted to measure client-centred attitudes (Jones 1963, Combs and Soper 1963, Porter 1950). The test-retest reliability of the scale was found to range from 0.88 to 0.91 for three different groups of respondents (Nelson-Jones and Patterson 1975). The issue of validity was less clear in that Nelson-Jones and Patterson attempted to assess content validity by asking client-centred counsellors to complete the questionnaire. Whilst all of those counsellors achieved high scores on the questionnaire, some disputed the degree to which all of the statements reflected a client-centred attitude (Nelson-Jones and Patterson 1975). The questionnaire was used for this study with the permission of the authors and is reproduced in full as Appendix 2.

In this study, each nurse was asked to fill in the questionnaire. They were then asked to check the answers to each of the questionnaire items against the scoring system provided by the authors of the scale. The results of that scoring are said to reflect the degree or otherwise of the respondents towards client-centredness. Thus a score of 70 on the questionnaire (correct answers to each of the questionnaire items) indicated a extremely client-centred attitude according to the scoring system. Lower scores indicated a lesser tendency towards client-centredness. No problems were identified in administering or marking the questionnaire.

Analysis and findings

The range and mean scores were calculated for the total sample and for each of the sub groups. Figure 2.2 offers a comparison of the range and mean scores in each of the groups and the range and mean scores for the total sample.

The mean scores appear to fall into three groups :

1. Health Visiting Students, Professional Nurses and Community Psychiatric Nursing Students who all scored over 40 on the scale. These mean scores were are all beyond the mid point score of 35 in the attitude scale. It should be noted, however, that individual scores varied considerably within the groups.

2. District Nursing Students, Staff Nurses and Qualified Community Psychiatric Nurses who all scored between 35 and 40 on the scale. In these groups, one group had a mean score at the mid point of the attitude scale and the other two scored just over the mid point. Individual scores varied considerably.

3. State Registered Nurses and Practice Nurses who scored 33 and 31 respectively. (Figure 2.1). In these groups, neither mean score was above the mid point on the attitude scale, although individual scores, again, varied.

The picture to emerge from the group as a whole was that there was only a slight tendency towards a client-centred attitude (mean score = 39). There was, however, a wide range of scores achieved throughout the group.

Nursing Group	Sample Size	Range	Mean Group Score
District Nursing Students	24	24 - 47	37
Health Visiting Students	24	32 - 59	45
Staff Nurses	22	25 - 50	35
Professional Nurses	20	35 - 67	47
Community Psychiatric Nursing Students	21	24 - 63	44
Qualified Community Psychiatric Nurses	12	27 - 50	37
State Enrolled Nurses	10	27 - 45	33
Practice Nurses	9	22 - 37	31
TOTALS	142	22 - 67	39

Figure 2.2 : Comparison of Range and Mean Scores (n =142)

Discussion

Perhaps the most notable finding was the lack of a tendency towards client-centredness in the nurses completing this questionnaire. Given the increasing emphasis on individualised care (Sparrow 1986) the encouragement of patient autonomy (Meleis 1985), this is disappointing. It suggests that some nurses may still be more comfortable with an interpersonal style that is prescriptive rather than facilitating. At first glance, this may suggest that they could be comfortable with the style of counselling to be found in the AIDS counselling field.

However, some of the groups of respondents showed tendencies towards a client-centred approach. Notably, the health visiting students, professional nurses and community psychiatric nursing students showed more of a tendency in this direction than did other groups. Whilst it may be the case that professional nurses, through their increased nursing experience have come to value a less directive approach, the student group findings are less easy to explain. One possibility is that students tend to discuss such things as interpersonal skills training as part of their courses and this may have influenced their completion of the questionnaire. On the other hand, if this is the case, it is difficult to explain why the district nursing student group did not score in a similar pattern.

It is notable that no particular difference can be noted between the scores of the general nurses and those of community psychiatric nurses and community psychiatric nursing students. It may have been imagined that psychiatric nurses, given the emphasis on interpersonal skills training prescribed by the 1982 syllabus of training (ENB 1982) would value the client-centred approach more highly.

On the other hand, it is notable that the community psychiatric nursing students scored more highly than their qualified counterparts. There are at least three possible explanations here. One is that the 1982 syllabus has affected more recently qualified nurses towards the client-centred approach. Another is that those students are studying interpersonal skills on their courses and are thus more aware of the client-centred approach. A third possibility is that such students are more idealistic about the nature of interpersonal relationships than are nurses in practice. What is noticeable from the findings is the tendency for nurses-in-practice to score lower on the attitude scale than those who are students (with the exception of the group labelled 'professional nurses').

The tendency for students of various sorts to score more highly than their qualified counterparts may also be accounted for in terms of their being in training and thus away from the pressures of the 'real world' of nursing. In the clinical situation, nurses frequently have to focus on getting through the work, whilst students may be able to be more reflective about what they should do in their relations with others.

Further, it is notable that the professional nurse group tended to score higher than other groups. Given that this group was made up of nursing managers, tutors and senior tutors with some experienced ward sisters, it is possible that their score on the scale has been influenced to a degree by the lack of clinical contact of some members of the group. Perhaps the more removed a practitioner becomes from direct patient care, the greater tendency they have to describe nursing actions from the 'ideal' standpoint.

The clinical component of nursing carries with it responsibility, the need to make swift and important decisions and calls for direct response to a whole range of human problems. The clinical practitioner is thinking on her feet, whilst students and those at one remove from the clinical setting can afford, and are encouraged to be (Ashworth and Morrison 1989), more reflective about the ideal role.

Also, two other points are relevant here. It may be that nurses who work under pressure and have to make many 'instant' decisions will also tend to be more prescriptive in their responses to others. It may be that the client-centred approach, is, by its reflective nature, more time consuming and therefore less immediately attractive as a form of nursing response. Nor may it be the most efficient way to work in busy clinical settings.

The second point is that because of the problem of having to respond to so many requests from patients, relatives and colleagues, the nurse may adopt a prescriptive role as a means of defense against anxiety, rather as Menzies (1960) described. This explanation may account for why the enrolled nurse and the practice nurse groups scored low in terms of client-centredness. Both groups have close contact with large numbers of patients and both work in busy (if different) settings. Arguably, too, the practice nurse group may perceive their role as being legitimately more prescriptive in nature.

All of these issues raise questions about the relevance of the client-centred approach in nursing. Whilst it clearly has a place in psychotherapy and counselling (Rogers 1967, Tschudin 1986), it may be that a variety of both client-centred and more prescriptive approaches to nurse-patient interaction are the norm. Perhaps, too, they are required in certain clinical settings. The study raises various questions about the nature of the nurse-patient relationship. More research remains to be done in this complicated field.

All of this has implications for nurses and AIDS counselling. If, as has been suggested by this study, nurses see themselves as more skilled in the prescriptive role than in the client-centred role, then they may well find that the information giving role that seems to be identified for the AIDS counsellor, may suit them. On the other hand, this presupposes a number of things. First, it glosses over the content and nature of AIDS counselling. It cannot be assumed that because nurses appear to be effective at being prescriptive and information giving that those skills will automatically transfer into the field of AIDS and AIDS counselling. Second, it presupposes that AIDS counselling will remain fairly prescriptive and information oriented. If, as will be developed later in this study, the role of the AIDS counsellor changes, it may be that the immediate call for information and advice as key features of the AIDS counselling role will be modified to include a more client-centred approach.

Personal qualities of the counsellor

Counselling, of the client-centred sort, requires at least two things : a) the development of certain personal qualities and b) the learning of basic interpersonal skills. Three clusters of personal qualities were identified by humanistic therapist and educator Carl Rogers (1967, 1983) as necessary and sufficient for therapeutic change in the counselling relationship. This is a particularly strong claim for Rogers to have made for, as we shall see, the qualities are open to interpretation by the reader, researcher or counsellor. Rogers three clusters of qualities were :

1) Warmth and genuineness,
2) Empathic understanding and
3) Unconditional positive regard.

Warmth and genuineness

Warmth, in the counselling relationship refers to being approachable and open to the patient or colleague. Schulman (1982) argues that the following characteristics are involved in demonstrating the concept of warmth : equal worth, absence of blame, nondefensiveness and closeness. Warmth is as much a frame of mind as a skill and perhaps one developed through being honest with yourself and being prepared to be open with others. It also involves treating the other person as an equal human being.

Martin Buber (1958) the philosopher and therapist made a distinction between the 'I-it' relationship and the 'I-Thou (or 'I-you') relationship. In the I-it relationship, one person treats the other as an object, as a thing. In the I-thou relationship, there occurs a meeting of persons, transcending any differences there may be in terms of status, background, lifestyle, belief or value systems. In the I-thou relationship there is a sense sharing and of mutuality, a sense that can be contagious and is of particular value in AIDS counselling.

What is not clear is the degree to which a counselling-client relationship can be a mutual relationship. Rogers (1967) argues that the relationship can be a mutual one but Buber acknowledges that because it is always the client who seeks out the professional and comes to that professional with problems, the relationship is, necessarily, unequal and lacking in mutuality. For Buber, the professional relationship starts and progresses from an unequal footing:

> He comes for help to you. You don't come for help to him. And not only this, but you are able, more or less to help him...You are, of course, a very important person for him. But not a person whom he wants to see and to know and is able to. He is floundering around, he comes to you. He is, may I say, entangled in your life, in your thoughts, in your being, your communication, and so on. But he is not interested in you as you. It cannot be. (Buber 1966).

Thus warmth must be offered by the counsellor but the feeling may not necessarily be reciprocated by the client. There is, as well, another problem with the notion of warmth. We all perceive personal qualities in different sorts of ways. One person's warmth is another person's sickliness or sentimentality. We cannot guarantee how our 'warmth' will be perceived by the other person. In a more general way, however, 'warmth' may be compared to 'coldness'. It is clear that the 'cold' person would not be the ideal person to undertake helping another person in a counselling setting! It is salutary, however, to reflect on the degree to which there are 'cold' people working in the counselling arena and to question why this may be so. It is possible that interpersonal skills training may help this situation for it may be that some 'cold' people are unaware of their coldness.

To a degree, however, our relationships with others tend to be self-monitoring. To a degree, we anticipate, as we go on with a relationship, the effect we are having on others and modify our presentation of self accordingly. Thus we soon get to know if our 'warmth' is too much for the patient or colleague or is being perceived by him in a negative way. This ability to constantly monitor ourselves and our relationships is an important part of the process of developing interpersonal and counselling skills.

Genuineness, too, is another important aspect of the relationship. In one sense, the issue is black or white. We either genuinely care for the person in front of us or we do not. We cannot easily fake professional interest. We must be interested. Some people, however, will interest us more than others. Often, those clients who remind us of our own problems or our own personalities will interest us most of all. This is not so important as our having a genuine interest in the fact that the relationship is happening at all.

On the surface of it, there may appear to be a conflict between the concept of genuineness and the self-monitoring alluded to, above. Self-monitoring may be thought of as 'artificial' or contrived and therefore not genuine. The 'genuineness', discussed here, relates to the counsellor's interest in the human relationship that is developing between the two people. Any ways in which that relationship can be enhanced must serve a valuable purpose. It is quite possible to be 'genuine' and yet aware of what is happening : genuine and yet committed to increasing interpersonal competence.

Empathic understanding

Empathy is a relatively new term, apparently coined by Titchner in 1909 to translate the German term 'Einfuhlung' (Bateson and Coke 1981). The term is usually used to convey the idea of the ability to enter the perceptual world of the other person : to see the world as they see it. It also suggests an ability to convey this perception to the other person. Kalisch (1971) defines empathy as 'the ability to perceive accurately the feelings of another person and to communicate this understanding to him'.

Empathy is different to sympathy. Sympathy suggests 'feeling sorry' for the other person or, perhaps, identifying with how they feel. If a person sympathises they imagine themselves as being in the other person's position. With empathy the person tries to imagine how it is to be the other person. Feeling sorry for that person does not really come into it. Being empathic, says Rogers:

> ...means entering the private perceptual world of the other and becoming thoroughly at home in it. It involves being sensitive, moment to moment, to the changing felt meanings which flow in

this other person, to the fear or rage or tenderness or confusion or whatever... (Rogers 1967)

Gerard Egan (1990) offers a useful summary of the way in which empathy can be useful in the counselling or helping relationship. He suggests that empathy can :

- Build the relationship,
- Stimulate self-exploration,
- Check understandings,
- Provide support,
- Lubricate communication,
- Focus attention,
- Restrain the helper,
- Pave the way. (Egan 1990).

The process of developing empathy involves something of an act of faith. When we empathise with another person, we cannot know what the outcome of that empathising will be. If we pre-empt the outcome of our empathising, we are already not empathising - we are thinking of solutions and of ways of influencing the client towards a particular goal that we have in mind. The process of empathising involves entering into the perceptual world of the other person without, necessarily knowing where that process will lead to.

Developing empathic understanding is the process of exploring the client's world, with the client, neither judging nor necessarily offering advice. Perhaps it can be achieved best through the process of carefully attending and listening to the other person and, perhaps, by use of the skills known as 'reflection' which is discussed in a later chapter of this book. It is also a 'way of being', a disposition towards the client, a willingness to explore the other person's problems and to allow the other person to express themselves fully. Again, as with all aspects of the 'client-centred' approach to caring, the empathic approach is underpinned by the idea that it is the client, in the end, who will find their own way through and will find their own answers to their problems in living. To be empathic is to be a fellow traveller, a friend to the person as they undertake the search. Empathic understanding, then, invokes the notion of 'befriending'.

There are, of course, limitations to the degree to which we can truly empathise. Because we all live in different 'worlds' based on our particular culture, education, physiology, belief systems and so forth, we all view that world slightly differently. Thus, to truly empathise with another person would involve actually becoming that other person! We can, however, strive to get as close to the perceptual world of the other by listening and attending and by suspending judgement. We can also learn to forget ourselves, temporarily and give ourselves as completely as we can to the other person. There is an interesting paradox involved here. First, we need self-awareness to enable us to develop empathy. Then we need to forget ourselves in order to truly give our empathic attention to the other person.

Driscoll (1984) also warns of the limits of empathy when he writes:

> Showing that we understand should not be seen as incompatible in any way with any of the range of further interventions. The sequencing of therapeutic interventions is important. One who acknowledges another's position is more easily seen as an ally, and is in a better position from there to challenge and restructure. Expressing an understanding is thus an initial intervention which prepares the groundwork for later, more forceful strategies for change. In general, as each issue is introduces, we should convey that we understand the client's position on that issue, and then continue from there to interpretation and redirection.The empathic response is given an exalted position in classical client-centred counselling : it is the answer to everything, and anything else a counsellor might do is just plain wrong. Most eclectics use empathic responses but reject the restrictive ideology. We see the empathic response as but one of a range of available therapeutic responses (Driscoll 1984).

Driscoll views the concept of empathy as being bound up very closely with the notion of client-centred counselling and argues for a more wide ranging approach to counselling. In AIDS counselling, both from the point of view of the literature on the topic and from the research described in this report, it would seem that a more varied approach than just the client-centred is appropriate and necessary.

Unconditional positive regard

Carl Roger's phrase 'unconditional positive regard' (Rogers 1967),conveys a particularly important predisposition towards the client, by the counsellor. Rogers also called it 'prizing' or even just 'accepting'. It means that the client is viewed with dignity and valued as a worthwhile and positive human being. The 'unconditional' prefix refers to the idea that such regard is offered without any preconditions. Often in relationships, some sort of reciprocity is demanded : I will like you (or love you) as long as you return that liking or loving. Roger's is asking that the feelings that the counsellor holds for the client should be undemanding and not requiring reciprocation.

There is a suggestion of an inherent 'goodness' within the client, bound up in Roger's notion of unconditional positive regard. This notion of persons as essentially good can be traced back, at least to Rousseau's 'Emile' and is philosophically problematic. Arguably, notions such as 'goodness' and 'badness' are social constructions and to argue that a person is born good or bad is fraught. However, as a practical starting point in the counselling relationship, it seems to be a good idea that we assume an inherent, positive and life-asserting characteristic in the client. It seems difficult to argue otherwise. It would be odd, for instance, to engage in the process of counselling with the view that the person was essentially bad, negative and unlikely to grow or develop!

Unconditional positive regard, then, involves a deep and positive feeling for the other person, perhaps equivalent, in the health professions to what Alistair Campbell has called 'moderated love' (Campbell 1984). He talks of 'lovers and professors', suggesting that certain professionals profess to love, thus claiming both the ability to be professional and to express altruistic love or disinterested love for others. It is interesting that Campbell seems to be suggesting that a counselling professional can 'professionally care' or even 'professionally love' her client.

Other characteristics of the effective counsellor

Drawing on the work of Ornstein (1975), Mayeroff (1971) and others, other characteristics of the effective counsellor may be identified.

Intuition

Intuitive is perhaps the most undervalued of personal qualities. Intuition refers to knowledge and insight that arrives independently of the senses. In other words we just 'know'. Ornstein (1975) who studies the literature on the differences between the two sides of the brain identified intuition with the right side. He argued that the tow sides have qualitatively different functions. The left side is concerned with cognitive processes and with rationality. The right is more to do with holism, creativity and intuition, according to Ornstein. If he is right, the implication is that if the intuitive aspect is developed further (along with creativity) then both sides of the brain will function optimally. Ornstein argues that the present Western culture is dominated by the left brain approach to education and development. He calls for an educational system that honours creativity and intuition alongside the development of rationality.

Perhaps we neglect intuition through fear of it or concern that it may not be trusted. On the other hand, it is likely that we all have 'hunches' that when followed turn out to be 'right'. Many aspects of nursing require the nurse to be intuitive. Sometimes, in order to empathise with another person we have to guess at what they are feeling. Sometimes we seem to 'know' what they are feeling. Certainly, counselling depends to a fair degree on this intuitive ability. Carl Rogers, founder of client-centred counselling noted that when he had a hunch about something that was happening in a counselling session, it invariably helped if her verbalised that intuition (Roger 1967). Using intuition consciously and openly takes courage and sometimes it is wrong. One the other hand, used hand in hand with more traditional forms of thinking, it can enhance the nurse/patient relationship in a way that logic, on its own, never can.

Caring

In order to really help clients in counselling, we must care for them. Now this may sound obvious : after all, we belong to a caring profession. But what does it mean to care?

Milton Mayeroff, in an important analysis of the meaning of caring in human relationships (Mayeroff, 1971) describes caring as a process which offers people (both carer the and cared for individual), opportunities for personal growth.

Major aspects of caring in the analysis include : knowledge, alternating rhythms (learning from experience), patience, honesty, trust, humility, hope, and courage. Those elements are discussed in more detail here although the discussion is a little different to the one that

Mayeroff offers. The caring attitude is also discussed in a separate section of this chapter.

Knowledge

In order to care for someone, we must know certain things. First, we must know who they are. Think of a friendship. Friendships develop because as we learn more about the other person, we acknowledge that we like what we get to know. If we did not like it, the friendship would not develop at all. In the context of nursing, we must also get to know the patient in order to get to care for them.

In another sense, however, we need knowledge to use and to give to the patient. In the sense of knowledge to use, we need to know certain things about what is wrong with the other person in order to help them. Thus, in caring for a person with AIDS, we need to know various things about the nature of the condition.

It is worth noting, however, that there are definite limits to what we need know in order to care for others. We cannot know very much about what is best for the other person when it comes to their personal or emotional life. It is tempting, when someone has personal problems to offer them advice. Such advise is only rarely helpful. One moment's reflection will reveal the fact that each of us lives a very different personal life to the next person. Whilst as nurses we can all come to know something about the nature of diabetes, we cannot come to know very much about the personal life of the patient. When it comes to personal and emotional issues, the patient is the expert on his own situation. Caring, here, consist of resisting the temptation to tell the patient how to live his life or how to sort out his emotional problems. There are, of course, limitations to this particular notion of caring when it comes to AIDS counselling. As we have noted, the AIDS counsellor also needs to be up-to-date in his or her knowledge of AIDS and related condition. On the other hand, of course, no one counsellor is every going to be fully up-to-date in this way for the field continues to change so rapidly.

Alternating rhythms

Consider any relationship that you have with another person, whether in the family, with friends or with colleagues. In all these different situations, the intensity of the relationship fluctuates. Sometimes we feel very close to the other person, sometimes we feel quite distant. According to Meyeroff, this is an example of the 'alternating rhythms' of any caring relationship. No relationship (and that includes one with a patient) can stay intense and close for any length of time. There seems to be a natural cycle in the caring relationship - what may be described as the waxing and waning of it.

There is another sense of the term 'alternating rhythms'. This is the idea that we may have to continuously modify the ways in which we react with another person. Sometimes, one approach works. On another occasion, another is required. People vary from day to day. What works with them one day does not necessarily work with them on another.

If this is the case, then each new meeting with a person involves us reknowing them, with meeting them afresh. Thus, in the context of caring, we must learn this process of remeeting and reknowing the person for whom we care.

Patience

Caring for another person involves taking your time. Whilst we may hope that a relationship could 'warm up' quickly, very often other people take time to get to know us and to 'allow' the other person to care for them. Again, think of a close emotional relationship that you have with a friend. That relationship did not come about overnight. It took time for both of you to get to know each other and get to like each other. In this sense, then, the caring relationship requires patience. Caring relationships, whether with friends or with patients, cannot be rushed.

In another sense, too, patience requires tolerance. We need to appreciate that other people are not the same as us. We are required, therefore to accept the person for whom we are caring, 'warts and all'. We cannot hope that the other person will come to be like us. Such a position requires patience : both with the other person and with ourselves.

Honesty

Honesty is a positive thing. It is not simply a question of NOT doing things like telling lies or deceiving the other person but involves being open to sharing with them exactly how we feel. It involves being able to tell them the truth, whether that truth consists of factual information that they need, or whether it is concerned with our feelings for them. A prerequisite for being able to be honest with other people is being able to be honest with ourselves. A necessary requirement for being honest with others, then, is a degree of self-awareness, of being able to honestly appraise our own thoughts, feelings, beliefs and values. Put simply, if we do not know certain things about ourselves, we do not know that we do not know them!

Trust

Trust is a clear requirement for caring. Just as we have to learn to 'allow' a child to find things out for himself and to make mistakes for himself, so, with adults we must be able to trust them to learn from their own experience, to make decisions for themselves and so forth. It is easy for us, as nurses, to become 'compulsive carers' : we smother the person for whom we are caring because we cannot trust them to take care of themselves. Trust, then, also involves 'letting go'. It involves an element of risk taking and accepting that other people find things out in their own way and live their lives differently to us. Often, mistrust in other people demonstrates a distrust of ourselves. In the context of AIDS, trust in the relationship is essential. We trust others more when we are secure in ourselves. Thus, again, the need for self-awareness and self exploration.

Humility

To care for another person is a great honour. If another person trusts themselves to us, we need to be aware of the great responsibility that this involves. We cannot afford to become too flattered by the other person turning to us for care. We need to stay humble and to appreciate our own inadequacies and limitations.

If we are not humble, we are likely to feel an overvalued sense of our own knowledge and views. To be humble, however, suggests that we have much more to learn. In the caring relationship, if we stay humble we stay open to new learning and to finding out more about the other person. Also, in AIDS counselling, humility is essential given the little we know about the hope of a cure.

We need to remain humble about the degree to which we can help people at all. Counselling does not offer all the answers and we must be reserved about our successes. The true test of counselling is whether or not the client does anything as a result of our counselling. The talking part is easy : it is the changing that is difficult.

Hope

To care for another person is to affirm that we believe in their ability to overcome problems and adversity. We cannot care without hope. If we do, we may just as well abandon the whole enterprise, for why are we bothering to care at all?

To counsel at all, suggests hope. As we grow fond of someone (which is often, though not always, the outcome of caring) we want to know them more and expect to see more of them. If we do not have hope, then we cannot expect this desire to be fulfilled. In the end, we would not enter into a counselling relationship if we really thought that we had no hope, either for ourselves or for the person with whom we were counselling. One of the issues that respondents in this study frequently referred to was the problem of maintaining optimism in AIDS counselling given the lack of cure and the typical course of the disease. Injecting hope into the AIDS counselling relationship seems to be a vital aspect of that relationship.

Courage

A lot is at stake when we care for someone else. Despite our efforts, despite our hope, they may not recover or, less dramatically, they may not care for us. They may not even like us! Thus to care is something of a gamble. Just as we cannot know the future, we cannot anticipate the outcome of our caring. Thus to care takes considerable courage.

It takes courage, too, to share ourselves with another person. Whilst caring may not always be a reciprocal relationship, it is likely that we will need to give of ourselves in the caring role. We may also need to tell the person for whom we are caring things about ourselves. As you tell me about you, the unwritten rule is that I tell you about me.

In this sense, caring is a process of 'coming to know' the other person. This sharing of self takes courage. We are all vulnerable and all fear that our self-disclosure may not be accepted by the other person. Usually, of course, it is. There are occasions when it will not be. It is for such occasions that we need to have a reserve of courage. This is particularly pertinent in the field of AIDS counselling where the client may find he or she experiences a change of self-preception as a result of knowing that he or she has AIDS.

These are some of the clements involved in caring for another person. It is not an exhaustive account and often a rather abstract one. Also, it is quite possible to add to Mayeroff's list of aspects of caring in such a way as to highlight a certain arbitrariness in his selection. Suffice to say, though, that unless we care for the client, we are unlikely to be very successful in our counselling.

Caring attitude

An essential component of the counselling relationship, in AIDS counselling as in other sorts, is the notion of caring. Morrison (1989, 1990, 1991) has described what he calls the caring attitude : an attitude made up of a variety of themes which attempt to capture the essence of caring in a professional context. The themes that contribute to Morrison's idea of a caring attitude are :

- personal qualities,
- clinical work style,
- interpersonal approach,
- concern for others,
- level of motivation,
- use of time (Morrison 1991).

These themes seem to move away from the abstract discussion of what it means to care for another person in a therapuetic relationship and begin to offer practical and behavioural indicators of what makes up a caring relationship with another person - particularly in the context of nursing. It is only recently that the whole notion of caring has begun to be researched in a professional context (Watson 1985, Leininger 1988). Many of the important issues have yet to be addressed, such as :

- The inherent contradiction of having 'professional carers',

- The question of power and control in the counselling and caring relationship,
- The 'lived experience' of caring and being cared for,
- Varieties of caring in different clinical and social settings,
- The similarities between formal and informal care,
- The political relationship between the organisation and the individual carer,
- The perception of people with AIDS to those who care for them and vice versa,
- The role of the professional in caring for the person with AIDS.

Further research in all of these areas can only help in the improvement of the care and counselling that is offered people with AIDS. We still have a considerable way to go in order to be clear about what does and does not help another person in a caring relationship.

Sense of humour

Humour plays a part in most people's lives. Whilst it is not an immediately obvious quality for the counselling, I believe that it is an important one. Humour has an almost universal power to defuse tension, relieve stress and bring a sense of perspective to a situation. It is as thought if we can laugh at ourselves, we get a view of the real size of the problem. Helping people to gently laugh at themselves can be therapeutic. That is not to say that the counsellor should in any way be fatuous, ridiculing or sarcastic - far from it. Suffice to say that small doses of gentle humour can make all the difference to effective counselling. On the other hand, the counsellor who is too earnest and humourless is one who can often appear inhuman and of no real value to the client. The psychologist, Carl Jung, once noted that the person who has lost his of her sense of humour has lost an important aspect of their spiritual make up.

Arnold and Boggs note the following variables that contribute to the successful use of humour as a communication strategy :

- knowledge of the client's response pattern,
- an overly intense situation,
- timing,
- the client's developmental level (Arnold and Boggs 1989).

In other words, we need to know something about the client's own sense of humour, we can use humour to take the sting out of a situation, we need to time our use of humour carefully and we need to be aware of the client's ability to appreciate our use of humour. As Synder (1985) noted, many studies have noted how idiosyncratic humour is : what I find funny, you may not.

A sense of the tragic

This is almost the opposite pole of the previous quality. All counsellors need to be acutely aware of people's ability to experience tragedy . The Buddhist faith notes one central truth : that all life is suffering. The sense of the tragic is an acknowledgement of the tragic aspects of life : the 'unreasonableness' of much of what happens to us, the arbitrariness of much of life and so on. Without a sense of the tragic and of other people's ability to experience tragedy, we are likely to take only a superficial view of other people's suffering. This can produce stilted and unhelpful responses such as the following :

> 'Don't worry. I'm sure its not as bad as you think. It'll all work out in the end.'

A balance between, on the one hand, having a sense of humour and, on the other, having a profound sense of the tragic is an ideal one for the counsellor. In a sense, the two are complimentary, for, almost paradoxically, both contain elements of the other. The most tragic situation can have humorous elements to it : some humour is also tragic.

Self-awareness

Self-awareness is the process of getting to know yourself better. A considerable literature has been generated on the topic and the reader is referred to that for a more detailed analysis of the notion (Bond 1986, Burnard 1990, Arnold and Boggs 1989) Summarising the literature on the topic, it is possible to suggest that self-awareness in counselling is helpful for the following reasons :

- it helps you to avoid confusing your problems with the client's problems. Without awareness, it is often easy to confuse our 'ego boundaries' with those of the other person. That is to say that it is easy to lose sight of what we think and what the other person thinks. As an example of how this happens, try to recall when you were under the influence of someone who had a stronger personality than you. When this happened, it was probably difficult to know whether some of the things you thought were 'your' thoughts or the thoughts of the other person. Without clear ego boundaries, we are often easily influenced by what other say and loose sight of ourselves.
- it allows you to work through periods of personal stress. Self-awareness helps you to appreciate and understand your limits.
- it allows you to work intentionally. That is to say that self-awareness can help you to choose what you say and do in the counselling relationship rather than just allowing it to happen. With awareness, we choose : without it, we are not even aware of the choices we have.

Criticism of the client-centred approach

Client centred counselling was born of a particular time : the three decades following the second world war and ending in the 1960's. Since the '60's the world map has changed, there have been a variety of political and social upheavals in the Western world and views about what constitutes good counselling may have changed as well. In recent years, the client-centred approach has been called into question.

Rogers, the founder of the client-centred approach offered a very particular view of the human situation. He suggested, consistently, for example, that he believed that people are essentially 'good' and left to their own devices can make the 'right' choices for themselves (Rogers 1951, 1967, 1983). This point of view is summed up by Rogers as follows :

> ...the innermost core of man's nature, the deepest layers of his personality, the base of his 'animal nature' is positive in nature - is basically socialised, forward-moving, rational and realistic. (Rogers 1967 : 36).

This theme of inherent goodness can be viewed as a reaction to the Freudian view of persons as essentially bad and to the Christian ethic of people as essentially evil (Murphy and Kovach 1972). In Rogers' case, it is made clear in his biography (Kirschenbaum 1982) that Rogers, in deciding that people were essential 'good', was reacting to an early training for preparation to enter the Church. According to his biographer, Rogers as a young man came to question his religious beliefs and then to reject them, preferring to view persons' as both essentially good and as responsible, to some degree, for their own actions.

Writing of the development of humanistic psychology in counselling, Woolfe, Dryden and Charles-Edwards (1989) have this to say :

> The object of person-centred counselling...is to help the client 'to become what he/she is capable of becoming' {Rogers 1951}, or, to employ an even more well-worn phrase associated with Maslow, to achieve self-actualization {Maslow 1962}. These terms have a slightly hollow ring about them in the enterprise economy of the late 1980s in Britain, in which the division between the 'haves' and the 'have nots' is sharply apparent. Striving for self-actualization is easier if one is well-off, well-housed, has a rewarding and secure job and lives in a pleasant environment than if one is unemployed, poor, ill-housed, and lives in a run-down neighbourhood. Terms like self-actualization simply do not feature in and do not derive from the culture of the 1980s. (Woolfe, Dryden and Charles-Edwards 1989 : 10).

Howard made a similar point rather more directly when, discussing the changing needs of clients who seek counselling, suggested about counsellors that :

> It is time we shed our naivety and the 'syrupy' illusions of Carl Rogers and his many cohorts. (Howard 1990 : 15)

These writers raise important questions that relate to issues in this study. There have been considerable changes in life in the UK since the 1960's. The political climate has changed, employment patterns and patterns of health and sickness have also changed, some would say irreversibly (Bowen 1990). Ashton and Seymour (1988) sum up some of these changes as follows :

> Fundamental changes are taking place both in the way we view ill-health and the way as individuals, families and governments

response to it. In the United Kingdom ministerial reputations and careers are being made and lost out of the health-related issues of AIDS, drugs, heart disease and the environmental conditions of the inner cities. The once sacred National Health Service is under attack for failing to deliver the goods and the long assumed immunity to accountability of physicians is falling away week by week. In Liverpool, 26 per cent of adult men are unemployed and nationally the infant mortality rate has just risen for the first time in 16 years. (Ashton and Seymour 1989 : vii).

Ashton and Seymour begin to raise the question of whether or not the client-centred approach is appropriate in AIDS counselling. In the previous chapter, it was noted that education and advice both have their part to play in effective AIDS counselling. It was also noted that the concept of AIDS counselling involved a wide and divers range of counselling. Thus it seems likely that a more prescriptive approach to counselling may well be appropriate in the AIDS field. On the other hand, Rogers was not only advocating a particular set of skills or counselling interventions, he was also suggesting a particular attitude towards counselling which involved respect for the client, appreciation of their range of choices and the fact that it was the client who, in the end, made his or her decision for him or herself. This aspect of the Rogerian approach may still be appropriate in all types of counselling.

Murgatroyd and Woolfe (1982) note that approaches to counselling and caring for people with different problems of living are also changing. They suggest that there has been a move away from the client-centred approach of Rogers towards an interest in short-term, crisis-oriented counselling for which more directive, action-oriented procedures are usually advocated.

A number of commentators and researcher's have also moved away from the client-centred approach to counselling towards a more challenging one and see confrontation and challenge as an essential part of the counselling process (Dorn 1984, Ellis 1987, Ellis and Dryden 1987). Farrelly and Brandsma propose four 'challenge related hypotheses' for consideration within the counselling movement :

- clients can change if they choose,
- clients have more resources for managing problems in living and developing opportunities than they or most helpers assume,
- the psychological fragility of clients is overrated both by themselves and others,

- maladaptive and antisocial attitudes and behaviours of clients can be significantly altered no matter what the degree of severity or chronicity. (Farelly and Brandsma 1974).

In a similar vein, Howard, Nance and Myers suggest that action and challenge are an essential part of human makeup and that people have a 'bias towards action' which requires them, directly or indirectly, to:

- change from a passive to a more active state,
- change from a state of dependency on others to relative independence,
- change from behaving in a few ways to acting in many ways,
- change in interests - with erratic, shallow and casual interests giving way to mature, strong and enduring interests,
- change from a present-oriented time perspective to a perspective encompassing past, present and future,
- change from solely subordinate relationships with others to relationship as equals or superiors,
- change from lack of a clear sense of self to a clearer sense of self and control of self. (Howard, Nance and Myers 1987).

Given the subject of this study and the fact that many of the people interviewed about AIDS counselling suggested that people need advice and guidance as well as being allowed to find their own way, it is possible that a wide range of
counselling strategies are needed in AIDS counselling. Also noticeable in the AIDS counselling literature is a tendency away from association with a particular style or school of counselling :

> ...one thing that the term 'counselling', as we have used it does not imply is adherence to a specific 'school' or approach to helping people. Counselling in the context in which it is used in this book is not something which only trained counsellors can do, it is something which anyone who is working, in whatever capacity, with people affected directly or indirectly by HIV and AIDS not only can do by must do. (Green and McCreaner 1989).

What is less clear is why the assumption is made that adherence to a particular school also means that a counsellor must receive specific training. It is possible to argue that an untrained person could also still work within a style or school of counselling by reading the literature on the topic and applying it to his or her practice. It may be that AIDS counselling will develop into a more structured field and draw from specific schools of counselling as the AIDS issue continues to be a major one and one that affects more and more people's lives.

Qualities of the AIDS counsellor

As we have noted at various points throughout this chapter, AIDS counselling is different from other sorts of counselling in some ways and similar to other sorts of counselling in some ways. Green and McCreaner (1989) summarise the qualities of the effective HIV/AIDS counsellor as follows :

> The good HIV counsellor needs good interpersonal skills, an understanding of the social, moral, and ethical context of AIDs and the ways in which this affects people's lives, an awareness of the issues which confront those whose lives are touched by HIV, an understanding of the ways in which people can be helped, and an awareness of ways in which they can be hindered by the counsellor (Green and McCreaner (1989).

They also conclude that a good background knowledge of AIDS and HIV is also indispensable to the counsellor although, as Silven and Caldarola (1989) notes, no one counsellor can expect to stay completely up-to-date with the rapidly changing AIDS picture.

The AIDS counselling field

Aids counselling covers a range of different sorts of counselling and responds to a range of needs. Given the diversity of the field, it is difficult to make generalisations about who asks for such counselling and who responds. Green (1989), however, offers a useful list of characteristics of AIDS counselling as it applies in the UK and Western countries :

- Counselling tends to be carried out by specialist counsellors who are either committed to HIV/AIDS counselling or take it on as a part of their work in sexually transmitted disease counselling or in infectious diseases. Counselling and primary medical care tend to be carried out by separate individuals,

- There are well-established voluntary groups, often with telephone helplines, aimed at those who are particularly at rise or know themselves to be infected,
- Most patients are aware when they are at high risk because most cases of infection continue to be amongst fay me, intravenous drug uses and haemophiliacs,
- As a result of (3) most individuals who receive counselling come forward for it themselves. They have ready access to medical and counselling facilities on demand. Counselling can, therefore, be concentrated on a few sites,
- A lot of counselling work centres around individuals who come forward for the test of who have been diagnosed as having AIDS. (Green 1989).

One other thing seems to stand out in the literature on AIDS counselling when it is compared to the 'traditional' counselling literature. In the AIDS counselling literature there is (predictably, perhaps) a much greater emphasis on information and advice giving. Whilst it is clear that people need up-to-date and accurate information of the medical sort and they need help with a range of social and financial matters, they also need help with a range of aspects of emotional issues, ranging from coping with the realisation that one has AIDS to coping with bereavement following the loss of a partner. Whilst the literature does address these issues, when compared to the huge literature on these matters in other sorts of counselling fields, there appears to be a need for more work in these areas. In other words, whilst 'traditional' counselling has been largely client-centred', the literature would seem to suggest that AIDS counselling can quite often be 'counsellor centred'.

Hugman (1991) offers a sociological analysis of the issue of power in the caring professions. He discusses the inherent paradox between those caring professions which seek to professionalise, on the one hand and who, on the other, seek to offer a individualised, human relationship on the other. This may be a problem in the professionalisation of AIDS counselling. On the one hand, the apparent aim is to encourage the person with AIDS to live as fully and as independently as possible, on the other, this is all done within the contexts of the medical and health professions. Whether or not the medical and allied professions really can work on a 'human' scale is worthy of further debate.

3 Counselling skills

Certain, basic 'traditional' counselling skills may be identified, although as we have noted, it is the total relationship that is important. This is particularly true in AIDS counselling and many of the respondents in this study indentified the prime place given to personal relationships in helping the person with AIDS. Skills exercised in isolation amount to little : the warmth, genuiness and positive regard must also be present (Rogers 1967). On the other hand, if basic skills are not considered, then the counselling process will probably be shapeless or it will degenerate into the counsellor becoming totally prescriptive. The important issue, in AIDS counselling seems to be a balance between being facilitative and being prescriptive (Heron 1990). The term 'prescriptive', here, refers to giving advice and making concrete suggestions. The term 'facilitative', here refers to certain specific sorts of counselling interventions which encourage the client to talk and discuss his or her problems. In this chapter, traditional counselling skills are reviewed along with some of the issues related to counselling training. As is so often the case, the word 'counselling' means different things to different practitioners. On the other hand, a reading of some of the literature on AIDS counselling would suggest that when people write of AIDS counselling they use the word in a similar sort of way to others who write of counselling. In the end, counselling seems to be concerned with helping people through a one-to-one relationship in which one is put in the role of counsellor and the other in the role of client : one who is helping and the other who is being helped.

Counselling skills

Attending

Paying close attention to what the client is saying and listening intently to them are the skills most often associated with effective counselling (Arnold and Boggs 1989, Rogers 1967, Tschudin 1990, Heron 1986, Burnard 1989). The concept of paying close attention is sometimes refereed to as 'presencing' or 'attending' (Egan 1982, Carkuff 1983). Richmond, McCroskey and Payne (1987) suggest that eye contact is the central issue here and that it can be used to indicate non-verbally that the counselling interaction is about to commence.

Listening

Listening has often been identified as the key skill in listening (Tschudin 1990, Burnard 1989, Egan 1982, Carkuff 1983). Listening is the process of 'hearing' the other person. This involves, not only noting the things that they say but also a whole range of other aspects of communication : tone of voice, use of catchphrases, expressions and so on. Given the wide range of ways in which one person tries to communicate with another, this is further evidence of the need to develop the ability to offer close and sustained attention, as outlined above. Three aspects of listening can be noted . Linguistic aspects of speech refer to the actual words that the client uses, to the phrases they choose and to the metaphors they use to convey how they are feeling. Attention to such metaphors is often useful as metaphorical language can often convey more than can more conventional use of language (Cox 1978). Paralinguistics refer to all those aspects of speech that are not words, themselves. Thus, timing, volume, pitch, accent are all paralinguistic aspects of communication. Again, they can offer us indicators of how the other person is feeling beyond the words that they use. Again, however, we must be careful of making assumptions and slipping into zone three, the zone of fantasy. Paralinguistics can only offer a possible clue to how the other person is feeling (Argyle 1975).

Effective listening behaviours

Another consideration needs that is considered in the literature on listening is the behaviours the counsellor adopts when listening to the client. Egan (1986) offers the acronym S.O.L.E.R. as a means of identifying and remembering the sorts of counsellor behaviour that encourage effective listening The acronym is used as follows:

- Sit squarely in relation to the client,
- maintain an open position,
- lean slightly towards the client,
- maintain reasonable eye contact,
- relax.

All of Egan's suggestions about these aspects of listening are well supported by the research literature on the topic. A useful review of this literature is offered by Murphy, John and Brown (1984).

First, the counsellor is encouraged to sit squarely in relation to the client. This can be understood both literally and metaphorically. In North America and the U.K. it is generally acknowledged that one person listens to another more effectively if she sits opposite or nearly opposite the other person, rather than next to him. Sitting opposite allows the counsellor to see all aspects of communication, both paralinguistic and non-verbal, that might be missed if she sat next to the client.

Second, the counsellor should consider adopting an open position in relation to the client. Again, this can be understood both literally and metaphorically. A 'closed' attitude is as much a block to effective counselling as is a closed body position. Crossed arms and legs, however, can convey a defensive feeling to the client and counselling is often more effective if the counsellor sits without crossing either. Having said that, many people feel more comfortable sitting with their legs crossed, so perhaps some license should be used here! What should be avoided is the position where the counsellor sits in a 'knotted' position with both arms and legs crossed. There are also important cultural issues associated with the crossing and uncrossing of the legs. In some eastern cultures it is considered rude to cross the legs in company or to allow one's feet to point towards another person.

It is helpful if the counsellor appreciates that they can lean towards the client. This can encourage the client and make them feel more understood. If this does not seem immediately clear, next time your talk to someone, try leaning away from the other person and note the result!

Eye contact with the client should be reasonably sustained and a good rule of thumb is that the amount of eye contact that the counsellor uses should roughly match the amount the client uses. It is important, however, that the counsellor eyes should be 'available' for the client ; the counsellor is always prepared to maintain eye contact (Heron 1977). On the other hand it is important that the client does not feel stared at not intimidated by the counsellor's glare. Conscious use of eye contact can ensure that the client feels listened to and understood but not uncomfortable. Again, there are various cultural variables associated with the use of eye contact. Some cultures such as the Puerto Rican, Japanese and Indian favour a more limited use of eye contact in communicating with others than do some Western and Latin American cultures (Arnold and Boggs 1989).

The amount of eye contact the counsellor can make will depend on a number of factors, including the topic under discussion, the degree of 'comfortableness' the counsellor feels with the client, the degree to which the counsellor feels attracted to the client, the amount of eye contact the client makes, the nature and quality of the client's eye contact and so forth. If the counsellor continually finds the maintenance of eye contact difficult it is, perhaps, useful to consider talking the issue over with a trusted colleague or with a peer support group, for eye contact is a vital channel of communication in most interpersonal encounters (Heron 1970).

Finally, it is important that the counsellor feels relaxed while listening. This usually means that she should refrain from 'rehearsing responses' in her head. It means that she gives herself up completely to the task of listening and trusts herself that she will make an appropriate response when she has to. This underlines the need to consider listening as the most important aspect of counselling. Everything else in secondary to it. Many people feel that they have to have a ready response when engaged in a conversation with another person. In counselling, however, the main focus of the conversation is the client. The counsellor's verbal responses, although important, must be secondary to what the client has to say. Thus all the counsellor has to do is to sit back an intently listen. The temptation to 'overtalk' is often great but can lessen with more experience and with the making of a conscious decision not to make too many verbal interventions.

Use of questions

Two main sorts of questions may be identified in the traditional approach to counselling : closed and open questions (Quilliam and Grove-Stephensen 1991). A closed question is one that elicits a 'yes', 'no' or similar one-word answer. Or it is one that the counsellor can anticipate an approximation of the answer, as she asks it. Examples of closed questions are as follows:

- How long have you known your partner?
- When were you tested?
- Are you still depressed?

Too many closed questions can make the counselling relationship seem like an interrogation. Cormier, Cormier and Wiesser (1984) note that closed questions can arouse considerable discomfort in clients in counselling settings. Such questions also inhibit the development of the client's telling of his story and place the locus of responsibility in the relationship firmly with the client.

Open questions are those that do not elicit a particular answer : the counsellor cannot easily anticipate what an answer will 'look like'. Examples of open questions include:

- What did you do then?
- How are you feeling now?
- What do you think will happen?

The literature tends to support the view that open questions are more facilitative and more likely to encourage the client to disclose problems and talk about the issues that concern them (Arnold and Boggs 1989, Heron 1986, Egan 1990).Questions can be used in the counselling relationships for a variety of purposes. The main ones include :

- assessing the client's ability to articulate ideas,

- eliciting the client's thoughts without presenting the direction of an acceptable response,
- acquiring a broad database of information,
- establishing a milieu for true, two-way communication (Arnold and Boggs 1989).

Funnelling (Kahn and Cannell 1957) refers to the use of questions to guide the conversation from the general to the specific. Thus, the conversation starts with broad, opening questions and slowly, more specific questions are used to focus the discussion.

Reflection

Reflection (or 'echoing') is the process of reflecting back the last few words, or a paraphrase of the last few words, that the client has used, in order to encourage them to say more (Heron 1986). It is as though the counsellor is echoing the client's thoughts and as though that echo serves as a prompt. It is important that the reflection does not turn into a question and this is best achieved by the counsellor making the repetition in much the same tone of voice as the client used. Some writers suggest that reflection as a tool is most useful when it is used in a compound sentence that connects the feeling aspect of the conversation with the appropriate content (Carkuff 1983, Cormier, Cormier and Weisser 1984). Reflection of thoughts and feelings formed the basis of the client-centred or Rogerian approach to counselling (Kirschenbaum 1979).

Selective reflection refers to the method of repeating back to the client a part of something they said that was emphasised in some way or which seemed to be emotionally charged (Heron 1986, Burnard 1989). Thus selective reflection draws from the middle of the client's utterance and not from the end.

Empathy building

This refers to the counsellor making statements to the client that indicate that she has understood the feeling that the client is experiencing (Egan 1990). A certain intuitive ability is needed here, for often empathy building statements refer more to what is implied than what is overtly said.

Checking for understanding

Checking for understanding involves either a) asking the client if you have understood them correctly or b) occasionally summarising the conversation in order to clarify what has been said (Burnard 1989, Heron 1986). Rogers (1986) used the terms 'testing understandings' and 'checking perceptions'. The first type of checking is useful when the client quickly covers a lot of topics and seems to be 'thinking aloud'. It can be used to further focus the conversation or as a means of ensuring that the client really stays with what the client is saying.

Co-counselling

Co-counselling developed in the USA under the influence of Harvey Jackins (Jackins 1965, 1970) and, in this country, John Heron (Heron 1978). It has made its mark within the field of experiential learning. David Potts (in Boud 1981) has described its use as a learning tool in a university course and James Kilty (Kilty 1983) has suggested the use of co-counselling in student nurse training. It can be of particular value as a self and peer support system for health professionals working in clinical environments that are particularly stressful : intensive care units, children's wards, oncology departments, hospices, psychiatric units and so forth.

Co-counselling is a two-way process in which two people take in on turns to spend time as 'counsellor' and 'client', The client takes time to verbalise and talk through issues and problems from everyday life, while the counsellor gives her attention. The counsellor in this relationship does not act in the traditional counselling manner. In other words, she does not offer device nor attempt to 'sort out' the client. In this self-directed approach, the client herself learns to examine her own problems and to 'counsel herself'. Each individual normally spends about one hour in the role of counsellor and one hour in the role of client. In this way, true interdependence is established. Neither part is wholly dependent upon the other. Responsibility is shared, tough responsibility for working through problems remains firmly with the client. The counsellor may be invited to make interventions at the request of the client, according to a pre-determined contract established between them.

Co-counselling can be used in a variety of ways. It can be a means of de-stressing for health professionals working in areas of high emotional involvement. The process of verbalising pent-up feelings to another person in an understanding and confidential atmosphere can be very therapeutic. Co-counselling can also be used as a means of developing self-awareness through the process of exploring inner thoughts and feeling and particularly buried emotion. It can also be used as a means of practical problem solving, of talking out personal problems and making decisions about any aspects of the person's life.

Co-counselling training usually takes place through a forty hour training course, during the course of one week, over two weekends or through a series of eventing classes. Advanced co-counselling and co-counselling teacher training courses are also organised in colleges and extra-mural departments of universities.

Fig 3.1 is a simplified map of the theory behind co-counselling. This is necessarily a simple guide to the theory and the reader is directed to the recommended reading list at the end of the book for a more thorough explanation of what is involved.

The assumptions behind co-counselling are that people are potentially autonomous and able to exercise choice. Through the process of living, the individual experiences various types of stress which cause the blocking or repression of emotions. If those blocked emotions can be freed, then the person can once again be capable of making life-decisions and exercising freedom of choice. Co-counselling aims at enabling the individual to express that blocked feeling and thus become more able to charge of her life.

There are implications, here, for professional practice. As a general rule, we usually want to calm down people who are frightened, reassure those who are crying and stop people from expressing anger. Could we as health professionals be trained to <u>enable</u> people to express those emotions as a therapeutic human act? In the fields of health care practice the value of such an approach is perhaps clear : expressed emotion is presumably better than repressed emotion. Pre and post-operative situations, before and after childbirth, following bereavement : all these situations involve emotional experiences. Health professionals can be trained to help their patients to express those feelings freely rather than a) prematurely stopping them or b) feeling inadequate and unable to cope. Co-counselling offers one approach to coping with emotion. First, it enables the individual to experience their own emotional feelings and second, it trains people in handling other people's emotional release.

Co-counselling is a clear example of experiential learning in that it asks the individual to review past and present experience and to reconstruct their understanding in the light of the discoveries made. The co-counselling format is simple and can readily be adapted to a variety of learning situations in health professional education. A number of the exercises in Part Two of this book have been developed out of co-counselling training.

The co-counselling format can be modified in various ways. The simple pairs method can be used as an introductory activity at the start of a learning session. The group is divided into pairs and one person in each pair talks to the other about whatever is at the forefront of her mind. Her partner listens but does not comment. After five minutes, roles are reversed and the 'listener' becomes the 'talker' and vice versa. The pairs format can also be used to explore particular issues e.g. the role of interpersonal skills training in health professional education - any topic that is relevant to the subject under discussion. The format offers an economical and simple method of identifying a wide range of views, thoughts, attitudes and beliefs. It also honours the students views and is not heavily teacher-centred as are more traditional methods of teaching and learning.

It also offers an ideal relationship for people who care for or who have AIDS. In this study, a number of respondents identified the need for those who have AIDS to be counselled by other people who either had a thorough understanding of what it was like to have AIDS or who had AIDS themselves. The co-counselling format seems to offer an ideal opportunity for practising 'equitable' counselling.

1. People are potentially autonomous, self-directing, positive and able to exercise freedom of choice.
2. HOWEVER, people are subject to a variety of stresses throughout life : early childhood experiences, partings, bereavement, difficulties in relationships, spiritual doubts and so forth.
3. Such stresses cause emotions (e.g. fear, anger, grief, embarrassment) to become 'bottled up'. This bottling up stops the person from functionally fully.
4. Through talking out and through emotional release (trembling, angry sounds, crying, laughter), those pent up emotions may be released. Such release is therapeutic.
5. The effect of emotional release is that it generates insight and enables the person to think more clearly, to become less stressed, more autonomous and more able to take charge of her life. She feels less 'acted upon' and more able to exercise choice. She can be spontaneously, positive and life asserting.
6. Co-counselling training, through working in pairs, offers people training in : a) listening to and giving attention to others, b) reviewing and re-evaluating life experiences to date, c) the release of pent-up emotion (catharsis), d) handling other people's catharsis, e) problem-solving and life-planning skills, f) self-awareness, g) stress reduction.

Figure 3.1 : A Simple Map of the Theory of Co-Counselling

Counselling training

It seems reasonable to argue that counselling skills cannot be learned simply through a series of lectures. Given that they all involve interaction with another person, such skills need to be learned through interaction with other people - through experiential learning methods (Kolb 1984, Heron 1973, Burnard 1991). A wide variety of experiential learning methods have evolved out of the field of humanistic approach and which are used to teach counselling skills. All of those methods focus on the student or learner being offered an experience, followed by the reflection and making sense of that experience (Kolb 1984). McCreaner (1989b) has recommended the use of experiential learning activities in the field of AIDS counselling training. She also identifies a range of aspects that need to be addressed in AIDS counselling training :

- Basic facts and information
- Safe environment for personal exploration (e.g. as preparation for training in sexual counselling)
- Improvement and practice of communication skills
- Developing an awareness of patient's rights
- Improvement of teamwork and co-ordinated care
- Demystification of AIDS and counselling
- Review of professional practice
- Instilling a sense of what it is like to actually counsel and encouraging and directing personal initiative
- Breaking through professional roles to create greater responsiveness and responsibility
- Attitude change and behaviour (McCreaner 1989b).

In this section, some of the experiential learning methods that have been used in counselling training are examined, critically for their use in counselling skills training and the development of such skills in nurse education.

Pairs exercises

Pairs exercises, are often advocated for use in the development of counselling and interpersonal skills in nursing and the health professions (Tschudin 1986, Heron 1983, Burnard 1989). The usual format for the pairs exercise is that each person nominates themselves 'a' or 'b'. Then 'a' practices the particular skill (for example, using open-ended questions) in the supportive presence of 'B'. After a period in these roles, the two people swap round and 'b' practices the skill in the presence of 'a'. Afterwards, the group reforms and participants discuss their experiences.

An alternative use of the pairs format is for the pair in question to take a theme and for one person to discuss that theme whilst the other person listens. After a prescribed time, the pair switch roles and the listener becomes the talker and vice versa. After an equal amount of time in this second phase of the activity, the pair may link up with another pair and discuss the issue in a foursome. This method is called 'snowballing' by Jarvis (1984)

Structured group activities

Structured group exercises allow for counselling skills to be developed within a learning group. There are a number of publications describe a variety of group activities for enhancing interpersonal, social and counselling skills (Kagan, Evans and Kay 1986, Murgatroyd 1986, Burnard 1990). The idea of these activities is that the group undertakes an experience after which they discuss their thoughts and feelings about the experience and apply the new learning to the real or clinical situation. The adventures of this approach include the sharing of a common experience, the generation of a wide range of possible solutions to practical problems and the realisation of both the personal and the common nature of group experience.

Structured group activities as a form of experiential learning had been advocated by Marson (1979) as appropriate for the development of counselling skills in nursing. Bailey (1983) writing of experiential learning techniques in psychiatric nurse training argued that structured group activities were geared towards uncovering unconscious material for expression and resolution in peer groups. This suggests, of course, that Bailey treated as unproblematic (at least in that paper) Freud's notion of 'unconscious material' (Hall 1954) - an issue that has been highly criticised in recent times by Masson (1990) in his review of psychotherapy in general. Masson's view is that <u>all</u> forms of psychotherapy involve one set of values and beliefs (the therapist's) being imposed on another person (the client or patient).

Role play

Role play involves the setting up of an imagined and possible situation, acting out that situation and learning from the drama (Figure 3.2) (Van Ments 1983). More specifically, the cycle indicates that after a role play, a period of reflection is necessary, followed by feedback from other participants in order that new learning can be absorbed from the drama.

1. Setting the scene
2. Acting out the role play
3. Reflection and feedback
4. Integration of new learning from the role play

Figure 3.2 : The Stages Involved in Role-Play

The first stage of a successful role-play, 'setting the scene', consists of inviting a number of participants to play out a scene, either from their own past or one they are likely to encounter in the future. Scenes replayed from the past are useful in that the role play allows further reflection on those past situations. Anticipated scenes, on the other hand, allow for the rehearsal of new behaviour.

Once the 'players' have been selected, scenery and props of a simple sort are used to create the invoked scene, for example, tables and chairs, suitably arranged.

Once scenery has been set and roles cast, the role play begins. The facilitator acts as 'director' and helps the actors to fully exploit their roles. Occasionally the facilitator may stop the role play and allow a character to slow down her acting or take time out to consider how best to play the next part of the scene.

When the scene has been played out to the satisfaction of the players, the facilitator asks the players to reflect on their performances and those of their colleagues. Following a feedback period the role play can be re-run and new learning, gained from the feedback, can be incorporated into the new performance.

Role-play has been advocated for use in interpersonal skills training and in the development of counselling skills (Nelson-Jones 1981,

Burnard 1989), group facilitation skills (Heron 1989a), assertiveness skills (Alberti and Emmons 1982) and social skills (Ellis and Whittington 1981).

Apart from the use of role play in the development of interpersonal skills, it may also be used as an aid to developing empathy; to rehearse initial practitioner/client meetings; to develop interview skills; to practice public speaking or the delivery of seminar papers and as a problem-solving activity. In this later context, a problem situation is acted out with a variety of possible 'solutions'. The actors and the audience decide which solution feels best after they have completed the various role-plays. Richardson, Bishop, Caygill et al (1990) described an extended form of role play in which mental handicap nursing students were encouraged to play the part of profoundly dependent patients for a period of 24 hours, in order to attempt to experience empathy with such patients.

Role play has been widely advocated for use in the training of nurses and as an example of an experiential learning activity for the teaching of counselling skills (Wibley 1983, Heath 1983, Barnes 1983, McNulty 1984, Kilty 1983, Dietrich, 1978, Goble 1990).

Silven and Caldarola have recommended the use of role play in the context of AIDS counselling, particularly in a group context, as follows :

> Role playing can provide a forum for the counsellor to model effective communication and for clients to practice disclosing information about their antibody status in a supportive setting. Ofent the client's difficulty in disclosing antibody status to friends or family reflects problems with self-esteem associated with being seropositive. (Silven and Caldarola 1989)

Psychodrama

A variant of role play is psychodrama (Moreno 1959, 1969,1977, Blatner 1988) In psychodrama, a 'real life' situation that has been lived by one or more of the group members is re-enacted and then discussed by those actors and by the group. The above stages are worked through in psychodrama in much the same ways as they are in standard role-play. Slight variations in approach may be noted, however, and the following stages offer a more complete guide to the process of psychodrama:

1. the scene to be replayed is selected,

2. the main 'actor', who has described the scene to be re-enacted, chooses fellow actors, from the group, to play other parts,

3. the main actor briefs those actors about their roles and gives them a clear outline of what happened in the real situation.

4. the psychodrama scene is played out. As it is, the main actor may stop the action to suggest small changes in performance. The aim is to, as completely as possible, recreate the past scene.

5. the performance is then processed by the group of actors and ideas are offered by any 'onlookers'.

6. after the discussion, the situation is replayed as the main actors would have liked it to have occurred.

Again, psychodrama has been advocated for encouraging the development of assertiveness and counselling skills and communication skills (Siegel and Scipio-Skinner 1983, Reed 1984). Watkins and Addison (1990) described an extended version of psychodrama as a form or theatre for encouraging nurses to explore their relationships with patients. It has also been used for exploring group members personal and professional life problems (Gonen 1971, Rowan and Dryden 1989). Both psychodrama and role play can invoke considerable emotion in both players and observers (Logan 1971).

The founder of psychodrama, Moreno, was a charismatic person. Clare (1981) noted the numerous reports of Moreno's charismatic qualities and the dramatic and overwhelming qualities of trained psychodrama therapists. Clare concluded that :

> In therapy after therapy, from est to primal therapy, TA to Gestalt, one encounters the difficulty in distinguishing between faith in the therapist and evidence that the therapy actually works, that is to say, that it produces in the final analysis what it promises. (Clare 1981 : 109).

This issue, the question of whether or not therapies (and indeed dramatic experiential learning activities) are carried out by charismatic people whose charismatic influence is, perhaps, as influential as the therapy or educational experience, itself, is an interesting and fraught one.

Goble (1990) after reviewing the literature on psychodrama advocated its use as an experiential learning activity for the development of interpersonal and counselling skills in nurse education programmes. He also identified some differences between role play and psychodrama in terms of purpose, focus, emotional content,scenarios enacted and duration of activity (Fig. 3.3)

	ROLE PLAY	PSYCHODRAMA
Purpose	Training	Therapy
Focus	Professional	Personal
Emotional Content	Low	High
Scenarios Enacted	Usually future work situations	Private life : distant past/ present/ future
Duration of Activity	Usually less than 15 minutes	Up to three hours

Figure 3.3 : Summary of the Major Differences Between Role Play and Psychodrama (After Goble 1990)

It can be argued that almost all of the above training methods developed out of the humanistic school of psychology which was described and discussed in the previous chapter. One of the hallmarks of the humanistic school is its emphasis on the individual and his or her experience of the world. Also noted in the previous chapter was the fact that some counsellors are beginning to question the individualism of that approach and its applicability to the late 20th century. Given that AIDS not only affects individuals but also partners and families and given that AIDS counselling may often involve more than asking the client to reflect on his or her experience (and may, on occasions, call for definite prescription and advice giving) it is possible to question the use of such training methods in the process of AIDS counsellor training. There are, perhaps, two issues here. The first is the use of the training methods themselves. It seems reasonable to practice counselling skills in the presence of other people and through the use of interaction group training exercises. On the other hand, the philosophy of individualism that has so far been associated with such methods does not have to be present in their use. It seems likely that a combination of interactive methods with appropriate didactic teaching methods about AIDS is possible.

This chapter has reviewed some of the traditional skills associated with counselling and some of the training methods used to develop such skills. The next chapter explores the notion of emotional release in the counselling process.

4 Helping with emotions

A considerable part of the process of helping people in counselling is concerned with the emotional or 'feelings' side of the person. Clearly, in AIDS counselling, the emotional aspect of the person will be an important one. Sketchley (1989) notes that a wide range of emotions may be experienced by the person who is diagnosed as HIV positive, ranging from fear, guilt and apprehension to worries about the likelyhood of infecting others and for the future of relationships. In the U.K. and North American cultures, a great premium is paced on the individual's being able to 'control' feelings and thus overt expression of emotion is often frowned upon (Heron 1977). As a result, we learn to bottle up feelings, sometimes from a very early age. In this chapter, we will consider the effects of such suppression of feelings and identify some practical ways of helping people to identify and explore their feelings. The skills involved in managing feelings can be seen to augment the skills discussed in the previous chapter- the basic 'traditional' counselling skills.

Emotions and AIDS

Given that individuals vary in their response to life-threatening situations, it is difficult to generalise about the ways in which people react to the knowledge that they are HIV positive or have AIDS. George (1989), however, identifies the following emotions that he suggests are frequently associated with the experience of having AIDS:

- Shock,
- Relief,
- Anger,
- Guilt,
- Decreased self esteem,
- Loss of identity,
- Loss of a sense of security,
- Loss of personal control,
- Fear of what may happen in the future,
- Sadness and depressed mood,
- Obsessions and compulsions,
- Positive adjustment (George 1989).

Presumably, too, this list could be easily added to. It is notable that only one of George's items are positive and he suggests that positive adjustment to the realisation of having AIDS may occur with little intervention from professionals. This suggests that the AIDS counsellor may well have to face a wide range of negative emotions. It will be noted that many of the emotions discussed by George were also discussed by the respondents in the present study.

Types of emotion

The range of human emotion is vast, from suicidal and profoundly depressed feelings on the one hand, to mania and acute happiness and exaltation on the other. Any attempt to map emotions or draw up a schema is bound to fraught with difficulty. Heron (1977) distinguishes between at least four types of emotion, that are commonly suppressed or bottled up : anger, fear, grief and embarrassment. He notes a relationship between these feelings and certain overt expressions of them. Thus, in counselling, anger may be expressed as loud sound, fear as trembling, grief through tears and embarrassment by laughter. He notes, also, a relationship between those feelings and certain basic human needs. Heron argues that we all have the need to understand and know what is happening to us. If that knowledge is not forthcoming, we may experience fear. We need, also, to make choices in our lives and if that choice is restricted in certain ways, we may feel anger. Thirdly, we need to experience the expression of love and of being loved. If that love is denied us or taken way from us, we may experience grief. To Heron's basic human needs may be added the need for self respect and dignity. If such dignity is denied us, we may feel self-conscious and embarrassed. Very often, bottled up emotion is a mixture of anger, fear, embarrassment and grief. Often, too, the causes of such blocked emotion are unclear and lost in the history of the person. What is perhaps more important is that the expression of pent-up emotion is often helpful in that it seems to allow the person to be clearer in his thinking once he has expressed it. It is as though the blocked emotion 'gets in the way' and its release acts as a means of helping the person to clarify his thoughts and feelings. It is notable that the suppression of feelings can lead to certain problems in living that may be clearly identified.

All of these emotions are intimately linked with the experience of AIDS. The person who does not understand what is happening to him or who knows little about the disease will experience fear. And fear was one of the most frequently discussed emotions in the present study. Anger can also be experienced by the limitations that AIDS brings to the person's life. The issue of grief as part of the experience of having AIDS has been widely discussed elsewhere (Green and McCreaner 1989, Dilley, Pies and Helquist 1989) as are the questions of embarrassment and loss of dignity.

The effects of bottling up emotion

This section draws on some of the approaches to the suppression and repression of emotion that have been discussed in the literature. Arguably, the AIDS counsellor will need to develop methods of helping the client to express pent up feelings. The first stage in offering such help is to identify some of the effects that bottling up feelings can have on the human organism.

Physical discomfort and muscular pain

Wilhelm Reich, a psychoanalyst with a particular interest in the relationship between emotions and the musculature noted that blocked emotions could become trapped in the body's muscle clusters (Reich

1949). Thus he noted that anger was frequently 'trapped' in the muscles of the shoulders, grief in muscles surrounding the stomach and fear in the leg muscles. Often, these trapped emotions lead to chronic postural problems. Sometimes, the thorough release of the blocked emotion can lead to a freeing up of the muscles and an improved physical appearance. Reich believed in working directly on the muscle clusters in order to bring about emotional release and subsequent freedom from suppression and out of his work was developed a particular type of mind/body therapy, known as 'bioenergetics' (Lowen 1967, Lowen and Lowen 1977).

In terms of everyday counselling, trapped emotion is sometimes 'visible' in the way that the client holds himself and the skilled counsellor can learn to notice tension in the musculature and changes in breathing patterns that may suggest muscular tension. We have noted throughout this book how difficult it is to interpret another persons behaviour. What is important, here, is that such bodily manifestations be used only as a clue to what may be happening in the person. We cannot assume that a person who looks tense, is tense, until he has said that he is.

Health professionals will be very familiar with the link between body posture, the musculature and the emotional state of the person. Frequently, if patients and clients can be helped to relax, then their medical and psychological condition may improve more quickly. Those health professionals who deal most directly with the muscle clusters (remedial gymnasts and physiotherapists, for example) will tend to notice physical tension more readily but all carers can train themselves to observe these important indicators of the emotional status of the person in their care.

Difficulty in decision making

This is a frequent side effect of bottled up emotion. It is as though the emotion makes the person uneasy and that uneasiness leads to lack of confidence. As a result, that person finds it difficult to rely on his own resources and may find decision making difficult. When we are under stress of any sort it is often the case that we feel the need to check decisions with other people. Once some of this stress is removed by talking through problems or by releasing pent up emotions, the decision making process often becomes easier.

Faulty self-image

When we bottle up feelings, those feelings often have an unpleasant habit of turning against us. Thus, instead of expressing anger towards others, we turn it against ourselves and feel depressed as a result. Or, if we have hung onto unexpressed grief, we turn that grief in on ourselves and experience ourselves as less than we are. Often, in counselling as old resentments or dissatisfactions are expressed, so the person begins to feel better about himself.

Setting unrealistic goals

Tension can lead to further tension. This tension can lead us to set ourselves unreachable targets. It is almost as thought we set ourselves up to fail. Sometimes, too, failing is a way of punishing ourselves or it is 'safer' than achieving. Release of tension, through the expression of emotion can sometimes help in a person taking a more realistic view of himself and his goal setting.

The development of long term faulty beliefs

Sometimes, emotion that has been bottled up for a long time can lead to a person's view of the world being coloured in a particular way. He learns that 'people can't be trusted' or 'people always let you down in the end'. It is as though old, painful feelings lead to distortions that become part of that person's world-view. Such long term distorted beliefs about the world do not change easily but may be modified as the person comes to release feelings and learns to handle his emotions more effectively.

The 'last straw' syndrome

Sometimes, if emotion is bottled up for a considerable amount of time, a valve blows and the person hits out - either literally or verbally. We have all experienced the problem of storing up anger and taking it out on someone else : a process that is sometimes called 'displacement'. The original object of our anger is now replaced by something or someone else. Again, the talking through of difficulties or the release of pent-up emotion can often help to ensure that the person does not feel the need to explode in this way.

Clearly, no two people react to the bottling up of emotion in the same way. Some people, too, choose not to deal with life events emotionally. It would be curious to argue that there is a 'norm' where emotions are concerned. On the other hand, many people complain of being unable to cope with emotions and if the client perceives there to be a problem in the emotional domain, then that perception may be expressed as a desire to explore his emotional status. it is important, however, that the counsellor does not force her particular set of beliefs about feelings and emotions on the client, but waits to be asked to help. Often the request for such help is a tacit request : the client talks about difficulty in dealing with emotion and that, in itself, may safely be taken as a request for help. A variety of methods is available to the counsellor to help in the exploration of the domain of feelings and those methods will be described. Sometimes, these methods produce catharsis : the expression of strong emotion : tears, anger, fear, laughter. Drawing on the literature on the subject, the following statements may be made about the handling of such emotional release:

- emotional release is usually self-limiting. If the person is allowed to cry or get angry, that emotion will be expressed and then gradually subside. The supportive counsellor will allow it to happen and not become unduly distressed by it.

- physical support can sometimes be helpful in the form of holding the person's hand or putting an arm round them. Care should be taken, however, that such actions are unambiguous and that the holding of the client is not to 'tight'. A very tight embrace is likely to inhibit the release of emotion. It is worth remembering, also, that not everyone likes or wants physical contact. It is important the counsellor's support is not seen as intrusive by the client.
- Once the person has had a cathartic release they will need time to piece together the insights that they gain from such release. Often all that is needed is that the counsellor sits quietly with the client while he occasionally verbalises what he is thinking. The post cathartic period can be a very important stage in the counselling process.

- There seems to be a link between the amount we can 'allow' another person to express emotion and the degree to which we can handle our own emotion. This is another reason why the counsellor needs self-awareness. To help others explore their feelings we need, first, to explore our own. Many colleges and university departments offer workshops on cathartic work and self-awareness development that can help in both training the counsellor to help others and in gaining self-insight.
- Frequent 'cathartic counselling' can be exhausting for the counsellor and if she is to avoid 'burnout', she needs to set up a network of support from other colleagues or via a peer support group. We cannot hope to constantly handle other people's emotional release without its taking a toll on us.

Methods of helping the client to explore feelings

These are practical methods that can be used in the counselling relationship to help the client to identify, examine and, if required, release emotion. Most of them will be more effective if the counsellor has first tried them on herself. This can be done simply by reading through the description of them and then trying them out, in one' mind. Alternatively, they can be tried out with a colleague or friend. Another way of exploring their effectiveness is to use them in a peer support context. The setting up and running of such a group is described in the final chapter of this book, along with various exercises that can be used to improve counselling skills. All of the following activities should be used gently and thoughtfully and timed to fit in with the client's requirements. There should never be any sense of pushing the client to explore feelings because of a misplaced belief that ' a good cry will do him good!' The following methods are drawn from the considerable literature on the topic of helping people with emotional release (e.g. Ivey 1991, Burnard 1989, Heron 1977, 1986, Quilliam and Grove-Stevensen 1991, Stevens 1971).

Giving permission

Sometimes in counselling, the client tries desperately to hang on to strong feelings and not to express them. As we have seen, this may be due to the cultural norm which suggests that holding on is often better than letting go. Thus a primary method for helping someone to explore his emotions is for the counsellor to 'give permission' for the expression of feeling. This can be done simply through acknowledging that 'Its alright with me if you feel you are going to cry...' (Heron 1986) In this way the counsellor has reassured the client that expression of feelings is acceptable within the relationship. Clearly, a degree of tact is required here. it is important that the client does not feel pushed into expressing feelings that he would rather not express. The 'permission giving' should never be coercive nor should there be an implicit suggestion that 'you must express your feelings!'.

Literal description

This refers to inviting the client to go back in his memory to a place that he is, until now, only alluding to and describing that place in some detail. An example of this use of literal description is as follows:

Client : 'I used to get like this at home...I used to get very upset...'

Counsellor : 'Just go back home for a moment...describe one of the rooms in the house ...'

Client : 'The front room faces directly out onto the street....there is an armchair by the window...the T.V. in the corner....our dog is laying on the rug...its very quiet...'

Counsellor: 'What are your feeling right now?

Client: 'Like I was then....angry...upset..'

The going back to and describing in literal terms of a place that was the scene of an emotional experience can often bring that emotion back. When the counsellor has invited the client to literally describe a particular place, she asks him, then, to identify the feeling that emerges from that description. It is important that the description has an 'I am there' quality about it and does not slip into a detached description, such as : 'We lived in a big house which wasn't particularly modern but then my parents didn't like modern houses much...'

Locating and developing a feeling in terms of the body

As we have noted above, very often feelings are accompanied by a physical sensation. It is often helpful to identify that physical experience and to invite the client to exaggerate it, to allow the feeling to 'expand' in order to explore it further. Thus, an example of this approach is as follows:

Counsellor : 'How are you feeling at the moment'

Client : 'Slightly anxious'.

Counsellor : 'Where, in terms of your body, do you feel the anxiety?'

Client : (rubs stomach) : 'Here'

Counsellor : 'Can you increase that feeling in your stomach?'

Client : 'Yes, its spreading up to my chest'

Counsellor: 'And what's happening now?'

Client : ' It reminds me of a long time ago...when I first started work...'

Counsellor: 'What happened there...?'

Again, the original suggestion by the counsellor is followed through by a question to elicit how the client is feeling following the suggestion. This gives the client a chance to identify the thoughts that go with the feeling and to explore them further.

Empty chair

This is a method described by gestalt therapists. Gestalt therapy is a particular type of psychotherapy which encourages the noticing of moment-to-moment feelings and changes within the client by both the client and the therapist or counsellor (Perls 1973). This method of exploring feelings involves inviting the client to imagine the feeling that they are experiencing as 'sitting' in a chair, next to them and then have them address the feeling. This can be used in a variety of ways and the next examples show its applications:

a) Client : 'I feel very confused at the moment, I can't seem to sort things out...'

Counsellor : 'Can you imagine your confusion sitting in that chair over there...what does it look like?'

Client : ' It looks like a great big ball of wool...how odd!'

Counsellor : 'If you could speak to your confusion, what would you say to it?' Client 'I wish I could sort you out!'

Counsellor : 'And what's your confusion saying back to you?'

Client: ' I'm glad you don't sort me out - I stop you from having to make any decisions!'

Counsellor : 'And what do you make of that?

Client : 'I suppose that could be true...the longer I stay confused, the less I have to make decisions about my family....'

b) Counsellor : 'How are you feeling about the people you work with...you said you found it quite difficult to get on with them...'

Client : 'Yes, its still difficult, especially my boss'

Counsellor : 'Imagine you boss is sitting in that chair over there...how does that feel?'

Client : 'Uncomfortable! He's angry with me!'

Counsellor : 'What would you like to say to him?'

Client : 'Why do I always feel scared of you...why do you make me feel uncomfortable?'

Counsellor : 'And what does he say?'

Client : ' I don't! Its you that feels uncomfortable, not me...You make yourself uncomfortable...(to the counsellor) He's right! I do make myself uncomfortable but I use him as an excuse...'

The 'empty chair' can be used in a variety of ways to set up a dialogue between either the client and his feelings or between the client and a person that the client talks 'about'. It offers a very direct way of exploring relationships and feelings and deals, directly with the issue of 'projection' : the tendency we have to see qualities in others that are, in fact, our own. Using the empty chair technique can bring to light those projections and allow the client to see them for what they are. Other applications of this method are described in detail by Perls (1969).

Contradiction

It is sometimes helpful if the client is asked to contradict a statement that they make, especially when that statement contains some ambiguity. An example of this approach is as follows:

Client : (looking at the floor) 'I've sorted everything out now : everythings O.K.'

Counsellor : 'Try contradicting what you've just said...'

Client : 'Everythings not O.K....Everything isn't sorted out'...(laughs)...that's true, of course...there's a lot more to sort out yet...'

Mobilisation of body energy

Developing the theme discussed above regarding the idea that emotions can be trapped within the body's musculature, it is sometimes helpful for the counsellor to suggest to the client that he stretches, or takes some very deep breaths. In the process, the client may become aware of tensions that are trapped in his body and begin to recognise and identify those tensions. This, in turn, can lead to the client talking about and expressing some of those tensions. This is particularly helpful if, during the counselling conversation, the client becomes less and less 'mobile' and adopts a particularly hunched or curled-up position in his chair. The invitation to stretch serves almost as a contradiction to the body position being adopted by the client at that time (Heron 1977).

Exploring fantasy

We often set, fairly arbitrary, limits on what we think we can and cannot do. When a client seems to be doing this, it is sometimes helpful to explore what may happen if this limit was broken. An example of this is as follows:

Client: 'I'd like to be able to live more fully'

Counsellor : 'What stops you?

Client : 'Fear of the whole thing I suppose...'

Counsellor : 'What's the worst thing about your situation at present?'

Client : 'Not knowing whether to come out or not'

Counsellor:'And what would happen if you came out?'

Client : 'Nothing really, I suppose... I just get anxious...'

Counsellor : ' So nothing terrible can happen if you allow yourself to come out?'

Client : 'No, not really...I hadn't thought about it like that before...'

Rehearsal

Sometimes the anticipation of a coming event or situation is anxiety provoking. The counsellor can usefully help the client to explore a range of feelings by rehearsing with him a future event. Thus the client who is anticipating a forthcoming interview may be helped by having the counsellor act the role of an interviewer, with a subsequent discussion afterwards. The client who wants to develop the assertive behaviour to enable him to challenge his boss my benefit from role-playing the situation in the counselling session. In each case, it is important that both client and counsellor 'get into role' and that the session does not just become a discussion of what may or may not happen. The actual playing through and rehearsal of a situation is nearly always more powerful than a discussion of it. Alberti and Emmons (1982) offer some useful suggestions about how to set up role-plays and exercises for developing assertive behaviour and Wilkinson and Canter (1982) describe some useful approaches to developing socially skilled behaviour. Often, if the client can practice effective behaviour, then the appropriate thoughts and feelings can accompany that behaviour. The novelist, Kurt Vonnegut, wryly commented that: 'We are what we pretend to be - so take care what you pretend to be' (Vonnegut 1968). Sometimes, the first stage in changing is trying out a new pattern of behaviour or a new way of thinking and feeling. Practice, therefore, is invaluable.

This approach develops from the idea that what we think influences what we feel and do. If our thinking is restrictive, we may begin to feel that we can or cannot do certain things. Sometimes having these barriers to feeling and doing challenged can free a person to think, feel and act differently.

These methods of exploring feelings can be used alongside the client-centred interventions described in the previous chapter. They need to be practised in order that the counsellor feels confident in using them and the means to developing the skills involved are identified in the final chapter of this book. The domain of feelings is one that is frequently addressed in counselling. Counselling people who want to explore feelings takes time and cannot be rushed. Also, the development and use of the various skills described here is not the whole of the issue. Health professionals working with emotions need, also, to have developed the personal qualities that have been described, elsewhere : warmth, genuineness, empathic understanding and unconditional positive regard. Emotional counselling can never be a mechanical process but is one that touches the lives of both client and counsellor.

It is suggested that these methods can be combined with the more traditional counselling skills described in the previous chapter and with a more prescriptive approach to enable the AIDS counsellor to work with a wide range of techniques and skills.

5 Exploring perceptions of AIDS counselling

The aim of the study reported here was to explore AIDS counsellors' and health professionals perceptions of AIDS counselling. The study grew out of the researcher's previous work on counselling (Burnard 1988, 1989, Burnard and Morrison 1989, 1990, 1991) and out of a reading of some of the literature on AIDS counselling (for example : Bor 1991, Sketchley 1989, Bond and Rhodes 1990, Bor, Miller, Perry et al 1989, Dilley, Pies and Helquist 1989 Silverman, and Perakyla 1990). That literature did not seem to emphasise the role of the nurse in counselling people with AIDS even though increasing numbers of people with AIDS will be cared for by nurses. The study, therefore, also considered the role of the nurse in AIDS counselling as well as looking at broader issues.

The study was a descriptive one which involved both qualitative and quantitative elements (Bryman 1988). It was qualitative in that it sought to discover the perceptions of a range of people. The data that was obtained was analysed in both qualitative and quantitative ways.

Sample

The study involved a purposive sample of 21 people who were engaged in aspects of AIDS counselling or in training nurses in this field (Fink and Kosecoff 1985). The sample was thus a mixture of people who had direct experience of AIDS counselling and those who were associated with training and teaching nurses in this field. Some were selected because they were recommended to the researcher as people likely to have views on the training of nurses in the field. Others were approached, directly, by the researcher. It is important to emphasise that this was not a sample of AIDS counsellors only but a mixed sample of counsellors and health professionals working in the field.

The aim in selecting the sample was to continue to interview people until similar sorts of views and perceptions were being heard over and over again. Where non-probability sampling methods are used, this method has been recommended by Denzin (1970) as a means of selecting the appropriate number for a sample. The sampling does not end until new concepts and categories no longer appear (Burgess 1982). This state of affairs was achieved by interview 17 and 4 more interviews were carried out to ensure that saturation of this sort could be said to have been achieved. The profile of the sample, by occupation, is illustrated in figure 1.

Occupations of Sample (n = 21)	
Nurse/Midwife teachers	9
Counsellor trainers/facilitators	2
Practising nurses	2
Gay switchboard counsellors	2
AIDS counsellors	2
District AIDS coordinators	2
Priest working with people with AIDS	1
TOTAL	21

Figure 5.1 : Profile of the Sample, by Occupation

Method

The respondents were interviewed using a semi-structured interview process involving key questions (Youngman 1978). Those questions were of the type that could be elaborated upon by the respondents. Following responses to the questions, the researcher often asked subsequent questions to clarify a point or to develop a theme. Some of the interviews were carried out face-to-face and others were conducted as telephone interviews (Walker, 1985, Dillman 1978). Interviews lasted between thirty five minutes and one and a half hours.

There are precedents for the use of telephone interviewing as a research method in the AIDS field. Yelin, Greenblatt, Hollander and McMaster (1991) used structured telephone interviews to determine the extent of work loss following onset of symptoms, the interval between onset of symptoms and cessation of work, and the risk factors for work loss among 193 persons with symptoms of HIV related illness attending the AIDS Clinic at the University of California, San Francisco. Lewis and Montgomery (1990) used telephone interviews of random samples of Los Angeles primary care physicians in 1984, 1986, and 1989 and obtained information about their AIDS-related practice experiences, and sexual history taking. In the Netherlands, De Vroome et al (1990) carried out several telephone surveys regarding knowledge about using condoms as a method of preventing the spread of AIDS.

Method of analysis

All of the interviews were transcribed, directly, onto a double-drive, Epson Equity laptop computer, using WordPerfect or Galaxy wordprocessors. There are precedents for this approach in that many researchers have discussed note taking during, or even after, the interview process (Burgess 1982, Walker 1985, Spradley 1979). As with the more familiar method of noting-taking (involving pen and pad), this meant that the frequently used process of tape recording and then transcribing from the tapes was omitted. Whilst the researcher sometimes had to be selective about what was transcribed and what was not, in practice this proved to be a fairly straightforward process. It became clear that people tended to 'lead in' to their answers with expressions such as 'It seems to me that...' and 'I would think that it is the case that...' It was felt that some of these could safely be truncated and sometimes omitted from the transcriptions process and thus the 'essence' of the interviews was captured in full. Often such 'lead ins' seemed to be a method of enabling the respondent to think out their answer. The lead in served as 'thinking time'. Field and Morse (1985) note that every qualitative researcher has to make decisions about what to leave out of an analysis and about what is to count as 'dross' or unusable data.

Answers from all of the respondents, to all of the questions were entered into a free-form database computer program, Memory Mate (Fremont 1989). A free-form database program is one in which data can be entered in any order and without pre-planning of the 'form' of the data. Short notes as well as whole pages of data can be stored and retrieved. The value of such a program is that allows constant recall and comparison of data entries. It proved ideally suited to handling qualitative data. Details of the use of this database in the project are offered in the Appendix.

Levels of analysis

Figure 5.2 Illustrates the levels of analysis undertaken on the data. These start with a simple content analysis of words used during the interviews and go on to a detailed qualitative analysis of the data using a modified grounded theory approach (Glaser and Strauss 1964).

Ist level	Simple content analysis of words used by respondents
2nd level	Simple content analysis of phrases used by respondents
3rd level	Content analysis of themes discussed by respondents
4th level	Detailed qualitative analysis of data in the style of grounded theory

Figure 5.2 : Levels of Analysis

Initial content analysis of words

First, a simple content analysis of all of the words used by respondents in all of the interviews was performed. In order to do this, each transcript had questions and the research comments edited out and all of the respondents' responses were joined together to form one large file. The file was then analysed using the Shareware program *WordFrequency* which offers a simple frequency count of all the words in a document.

Shareware has a unique marketing strategy. A shareware program is distributed free of charge (although a charge is usually made for the discs and the handling.) The idea is that you first try the program and then, if you like it, you send away a registration fee to use the program. In the first instance, you usually have between 30 and 90 days to try out the program before you register it. Further, during this time, you are encouraged to make copies of the program for your colleagues and friends. Then, the same principles apply : they are allowed to try out the program and then send of to become registered users if they find it useful.

All of the 'gramatical' words such as 'the', 'their' and 'you' were removed and the lexical words placed in a rank order of frequency of use. This last function was carried out by the 'sort' feature of the commercial wordprocessing program, WordPerfect.

Content analysis by words alone offers a simple but crude view of the overall issues contained in the interview. The words retained after this analysis are offered in the next chapter and give an example of some of the issues that seemed to be talked about the most.

Content analysis of phrases

After the content analysis by words, a simple analysis of phrases was attempted by identifying commonly used phrases and identifying the frequency with which they were used in all of the transcripts. Again, this was a fairly crude and limited method of analysing data but it did highlight certain ways in which language was used by the respondents and some of their concerns. It has to be said that this was the least successful and probably least useful aspect of the analytical process.

Coding and further analysis

This section discusses the more detailed forms of analysis carried out on the data. First, a content analysis of themes discussed by the respondents was undertaken. Each question was coded. Thus all of the answers to the question 'What do you feel is the 'person in the street's perception of the person with AIDS ?', were coded 'C' and all of the responses to another question were coded 'D' and so on. This enable the rapid retrieval of all of the responses to any one question, in a clearly laid-out format. Also, all data 'items' could be searched for using either single words or strings of words. In this way, it was possible to interrogate the database in a variety of ways. A more detailed description of how a free form database program was used in this analysis is described in the appendix at the end of this book.

Once all the data were collated and explored in this way, categories were sought for in each question using the process know as category analysis (Berg 1989). Once categories were established, the data were sorted into those categories. Sometimes, it became appropriate to rank order the responses within a particular category and this ranking will be illustrated in the section on findings.

Checks for validity were made in two ways. First, other researchers were asked to review the analysis method and the category system that evolved and asked to play 'devil's advocate' by questioning both the process of analysis and the categories that emerged. Second, a number of respondents were asked to review the analysis process and the category system as it applied to their interview. In qualitative research it is essential that the researcher reports an honest account of what it is that respondents are saying and what it is that they mean by their utterances (Field and Morse 1985, Burgess 1982).

Overview of the research design

The descriptors, phenomenological and grounded theory may both be used to describe the general approach used in the later part of the analysis. These are forms of qualitative research and as such aim to develop theory inductively (Field and Morse 1985, Glaser and Strauss 1967).

Phenomenology attempts to describe a situation stripped of preconditions, values or beliefs. Oiler (1982) suggests that phenomenology represents the effort to describe human experience as it is lived. Its origins can be found in the work of the existential writers, particularly Husserl (1931) but also Heidegger, Merleau-Ponty, and Sartre, (Patka 1972, Macquarrie 1972). In this study, the aim was not to start out with a particular set of beliefs or theories about AIDS counselling (though, clearly, the researcher had these), but to examine and explore the beliefs and theories of others, whilst attempting to 'bracket' the researchers own beliefs and theories (Husserl 1931). The notion of bracketing refers to the putting on one side of any value judgements that one might have about the subject in hand. Husserl argued that such a process of investigation lead to a clearer perception of the matter under investigation. The degree to which it is possible to bracket one's own beliefs and theories remains open to question. Arguably, it is impossible to set them aside completely for they are the means by which we make sense of the world and by which we formulate the next question in the research process. A degree of detachment and ability to bracket was arguably possible in the present study in that the researcher was relatively new to the field of AIDS counselling.

If it were possible to engage in this bracketing process completely, then the researcher would be working in a theoretical void, with no means of making sense of what the respondents were saying nor any means of knowing how to proceed. Nevertheless, the attempt has been made to ensure that the researcher's own beliefs and theories colour the material to a minimal degree. Following Reason and Rowan (1981) the researcher wrote a paper outlining his own beliefs and values about the subject area before commencing work on the research project. Simon, Howe and Kirschenbaum (1978) refer to this process as values clarification.

Two other methods were employed to attempt to cut down bias on the part of the researcher. One was a conscious effort on the part of the researcher to constantly check his own tendency to 'lead' in an interview or to rush to interpret the data that were collected. By 'interpret', here, is meant any attempt to prejudge how the other person was using words or to 'make sense' of what they were saying in terms of a particular theory. Here, we run into linguistic problems and problems of 'personal' versus 'shared' meanings. On the one hand, we cannot suppose that other people are using words in a way that corresponds to a dictionary definition or a technical definition. As Wittgenstein (1961) pointed out 'meaning is use' : when a person uses a word, he does so according to what he believes it to mean. There is no guarantee that the meaning that he imputes corresponds to the meaning imputed by the listener.

On the other hand, if there was no occasion on which shared meanings were possible, we could not communicate with one another, for every word spoken by an individual would acquire a 'personal' meaning that was not comprehensible to another person. A sense of how this could feel can be gained when a person who speaks another language to our own (and which we do not understand) begins to talk to us in that language. Clearly, communication is considerably impaired. The only time, in such a situation, that we can guess at what the person is talking about is when he uses a word that sounds similar to a word in our own language. In that case, we guess at meaning, in order to try to make sense of what he is saying. So it is, to a degree, in everyday conversation. We are constantly (and metaphorically) asking the question : 'what does he mean?' If we cannot answer the question to our own satisfaction then we will find ourselves confused and unable to make sense of the conversation. Clearly, such a state of affairs calls for a theory of 'shared' as well as 'personal' meanings.

This, then, is the problem of shared versus individual meaning. The method employed in this study to attempt to deal with this issue was to frequently check with the respondent what they meant by a particular word that they used. Hinkle (1965) suggests that 'laddering' or the frequent use of 'why?' questions can help in this respect. This approach was occasionally used but a more frequent approach was to simply ask the respondent to explain how he was using a particular word. It is acknowledged that such an approach is hardly foolproof. Clearly, to ask a person, after the event, what he meant by a particular word is no guarantee that the definition that he offers captures the full sense of usage. To ponder on the meaning of a word or expression after we have used it may lead us to expand on our thoughts about that word or expression. It is possible, too, that we do not always know what we mean when we use some words. Sometimes we get to understand the meanings of words by using them first, by 'trying them out', in order to explore how we could use them in the future.

The second method used to attempt to check any tendency on the part of the researcher to colour data with his own meaning and belief system was to frequently check any analysis that was carried out with the respondent. Once an interview had been analysed and ambiguity noted, that analysis was discussed with the respondent to further check for clarity and for the capturing of individual meaning. It is asserted that this is in line with the phenomenological approach to research.

Grounded theory is a deductive approach to exploring and developing a theory of what is happening in a given situation. The basic principles of the approach were developed by Glaser and Strauss (1967) who suggested that, for too long, social scientists had tended towards the development of 'grand theories' that were not necessarily grounded in what was happening in the world. In other words, social scientists had tended to adopt a deductive approach : first they developed a theory about the social world and then they set out to test the degree to which that theory could be held to be true. Inevitably, argued Glaser and Strauss, the temptation (consciously or unconsciously) was to confirm and develop the prepared theory. They suggest, therefore, that the opposite approach be adopted : that the social scientist first goes out and explores an aspect of the social world, immerses himself in it and allows himself to discover what is there. Only after this immersion has taken place do they recommend that theory about the social world be developed and then that the theory should be firmly grounded in the data obtained : hence 'grounded theory'.

Glaser and Strauss, having spelt out their objections to traditional approaches to social science research are then less specific about how the grounded theory approach should be operationalised. A number of research studies (Pollock 1989, Melia 1986) suggest that those studies were carried out 'in the spirit of grounded theory'. Other commentators have criticised Glaser and Strauss' lack of clarity (Stern 1985) and given this disparity between the criticism of traditional research techniques and their description of how the problem may be rectified may lead to questions about the degree to which the grounded theory approach represents a discrete research methodology at all. It could be argued that the approach represents a prescription about how to do certain sorts of research, without that prescription having been fully worked out. This may not invalidate Glaser and Strauss' criticisms of deductive approaches to research but the issue of whether or not it is possible to do 'pure' grounded theory research remains an interesting question as does the degree to which grounded theory can be completely differentiated from other sorts of phenomenological and qualitative approaches. The question of whether or not there is a need to draw such definite lines between concepts may be answered by considering that if we cannot clearly say what the grounded theory approach is and how it can be operationalised, then we are likely to run into problems in, at least, the following areas : defending grounded theory as a research approach at all, addressing questions of validity and reliability, using the approach in practice, developing theory out of the collected data.

The method of analysis used in the present study was a modified form of the grounded theory approach in that the data was explored for recurrent and emergent themes, those themes were then grouped together and out of the grouping of issues and themes, a very tentative model of what AIDS counselling might be about was developed.

Qualitative and quantitative methods in social science research

There is considerable discussion in the literature about whether or not the differences between qualitative and quantitative methodologies are differences of fundamental philosophies or whether they are differences of method (see, for example the reviews in Bryman 1988, Leininger 1985, Van Maanen 1983). At the philosophical level it is argued that the quantitative researcher adopts the position of determinism : that the world is always and everywhere subject to causal laws (Bullock and Stallybrass 1977). If causality is a 'fact' about the world, then the way to explore that world scientifically is to collect, measure and count examples of things that happen in it as a means of developing theories and laws. On the other hand, the qualitative researcher seems to be arguing that our perception of what happens in the world is always dependent on a number of variables that colour our perception of it (for example, our physiological make up, our cultural context, our education, our belief systems and so on) : thus we cannot ever perceive the world 'as it is' but only 'as we believe it to be'.

Therefore, the idea that we can ever cleanly and objectively collect, measure and count examples of things that happen in the world in order to develop laws and theories is always problematic. The qualitative researcher therefore tends to adopt a relativistic position and denies the validity of the quantitative researchers' position. It remains an open question as to whether all researchers question the philosophical bases that their methods rest upon but it may be argued that our beliefs and theories about the way the world is will always fuel our actions. Indeed, Claxton, seems to be attempting to bridge the philosophical differences between the absolutism of the extreme quantitative position and the relativism of the extreme qualitative position when he suggests that,

> What I do depends on what my theory tells me about the world, not on how the world really is, (and)... What happens next depends on how the world really is, not on how I believe it to be. (Claxton 1984 : 17).

At first glance, Claxton's position seems to echo that of the theorists who argue that everything is relative and that we can, as William James would have it, only observe the phenomena, never the noumena (James 1902). Claxton, however, goes further than this in suggesting that the world 'really is' a certain way and that we can somehow make comparisons between what we believe to be true and what is actually true. This begs questions about how it is possible to know that the world 'really is' a certain way (for Claxton to posit the idea that the world 'really is' a certain way is to suggest certainty that the world 'really is' a certain way. Another position would be that the world may be a certain way but it may not 'be' any particular way at all). Claxton seems to want to have an absolutist world working away beneath the surface of our theories and beliefs about it. If he is right, then he may offer a key to a marriage between quantitative and qualitative methods.

If there are, indeed, two things happening : a world as it actually is and people in it that are viewing it and theorising about it, it would seem reasonable to combine both quantitative and qualitative methodologies. On the one hand, the quantitative methods offer a systematic way of classifying and quantifying the world, as accurately as possible. On the other hand, the qualitative methods offer a means of studying peoples belief and meaning systems. Thus, the argument is often developed that a combination of the two methods should be used. It is this position that is adopted in this study : both quantitative and qualitative methods are used, although the predominant method is qualitative. It is not intended that the differences between the two approaches (in practice) be rehearsed here : those differences have been explored in detail in the considerable literature on the topic (see, for example Cook and Reichardt 1979, Filstead 1970, Gaut 1984, Pelto 1970, Raggucci 1972 and Van Maanen 1983).

In summary, then, the researcher set out to both explore individuals' perceptions of AIDS counselling (the qualitative aspect) and also to identify whether or not there was some agreement over the ways in which AIDS counselling was perceived by groups of people (the quantitative aspect). In a sense, no research project can ever be purely qualitative : every qualitative researcher necessarily engages in some form of categorisation and quantification in order to present his findings. The only way of getting close to 'pure' qualitative research would be to present raw data and to allow the reader to make sense of it. Even if this dubious practice was engaged in, the reader would presumably then begin his own categorisation and quantification processes.

Price and Barrell (1980) and Barrell, Medeiros and Barrell (1985) offer precedents for the approach taken in this research project. They suggest moving from personal views of the world (in this case, via qualitative analyses of interviews) through to larger scale investigations to identify any tendency towards consensus of otherwise (in this case, via a secondary analysis of the interviews to identify the degree to which the perceptions of those interviewed are or are not shared).

6 The view from the counsellors (1)

The findings described here offer various views of the data. Figure 6.1. illustrates the levels involved in reaching the findings discussed, starting from a simple content analysis of words and progressing to a more qualitative analysis of themes in the style of grounded theory.

1st level	Simple content analysis of words used by respondents and frequency counts of words
2nd level	Simple content analysis of phrases used by respondents
3rd level	Content analysis of themes discussed by respondents and frequency counts of themes
4th level	Detailed qualitative analysis of data in the style of grounded theory

Figure 6.1 : Levels of Analysis

Content analysis of words

An initial frequency count of words in all of respondents replies in all of the interview transcripts was carried out. The method for doing this was described in the previous chapter. The following tables, figures 6.2. and 6.3 offer examples of words from that content analysis of words. The words that are left out of this table are grammatical words : prepositions, articles, pronouns, modal verbs and so forth. Words that were counted were lexical words : words that have a distinctive semantic content. Words were only included in this table if they had been used more than twice and all ambiguous words (in this case, words with two or three possible meanings) were left out as far as possible. An analysis of this sort and at this level is inevitably crude but it does help to illustrate the sorts of issues that were being discussed by the respondents and the sort of language they were using.

Notably high on this list of words is AIDS itself, words such as 'counselling, 'skills' and also 'death' and 'fear'. The list is useful for reviewing the sorts of words that were commonly used and those that were less frequently used.

Once the lexical words in the transcripts were identified in this way, it was possible to search for groupings of words into categories (Field and Morse 1986). The words were written onto separate cards and three people who were not involved in the research project were asked to sort the cards into 'categories' of their own choosing. This is an adaptation of the multiple sort, or Q-sort techniques (Groat 1982, Burnard and Morrison 1990). The sorters were then asked to explain how they had grouped the cards. After discussion with the three sorters, the following categories of words were identified. The categories were felt to describe the sorts of words that had been used and were exhaustive in that they were able to account for all of the words.

- Professional/medical Words
- Personal/emotional Words
- Educational Words

Figure 6.4. illustrates the words occuring in each of the categories and the number of words in each. In this analysis, the most frequent sorts of lexical words identified in the transcripts were professional/medical words (41%), then personal/emotional words

(38%) and finally education words (21%). It seems reasonable to assume that health professionals and counsellors will use medical and medically related words fairly frequently in talking about AIDS but it is interesting to note the similar frequency with which 'personal' words were used, possibly suggesting the need to focus on the personal and emotional in AIDS counselling. Figure 6.5 offers a further analysis of the occurence of the words in the various categories. It identifies the number of times words in the three categories occured throughout the transcripts. These figures were computed by identifying the number of times words in a particular category were used in all of the transcripts and then adding together these numbers for a particular category. This gave the total number of occurences of professional/medical, personal/emotional and educational words within all of the transcripts. These figures must be read with caution. In computing frequencies in this way, it is being assumed that the category system devised here is exhaustive and that the categories are discrete. It will be noticed, however, that some words could be counted in more than one category and thus the analysis can only be seen as an approximate one. Also, it could be argued that the word AIDS was used so frequently that it should be left out of the computation. If the word AIDS is left out of the computation, then professional/medical and personal/emotional words occur with the same degree of frequency in the transcripts (Figure 6.6). The figures, despite these reservations, do give an approximate idea of the ways in which respondents used particular sorts of words.

Word and Number of Times Word Used in Transcripts	Word and Number of Times Word Used in Transcripts	Word and Number of Times Word Used in Transcripts
240 AIDS	9 Death	4 Family
176 Response	9 Health	4 Psychiatric
137Counselling	8 Disease	4 Caring
96 Nurses	8 Empathy	4 Attitudes
71 Need	8 Help	4 Burnout
68 Skills	8 Knowledge	4 Transfusions
59 People	8 Gays	4 Education
52 Training	7 Involved	3 Confidentiality
45 Person	7 Problems	3 Taught
36 Trained	6 Feelings	3 Psychological
36 Counsellor	6 Control	3 Disorders
31 Fear	6 Specialist	3 Prejudices
31 Difficult	6 Social	3 Drugs
30 Counsellors	6 Workshops	3 Patients
27 Important	6 Dying	
25 Personal	6 Facts	
24 Setting	6 Drug	
24 Discussed	6 Judgemental	
22 Qualities	5 Sexual	
21 Work	5 Learning	
15 Information	5 Support	
13 Listening	5 Sexuality	
11 Nurse	5 Groups	
10 HIV		
10 Gay		
10 Feel		

Figure 6.2 : Examples of Words Used by Respondents, in Rank Order, by Number of Occurrences in Transcripts (n = 21 transcripts)

Word and Number of Times Word Used in Transcripts	Word and Number of Times Word Used in Transcripts	Word and Number of Times Word Used in Transcripts
Aids 240	Feelings 6	Psychological 3
Attitudes 4	HIV 10	Qualitics 22
Burnout 4	Gay 10	Response 176
Caring 4	Gays 8	Setting 24
Confidentiality 3	Groups 5	Sexual 5
Counselling 137	Health 9	Sexuality 5
Counsellor 36	Help 8	Skills 68
Counsellors 30	Information 15	Social 6
Death 9	Involved 7	Specialist 6
Difficult 31	Judgemental 6	Support 5
Discussed 24	Knowledge 8	Taught 3
Disease 8	Learning 5	Trained 36
Disorders 3	Listening 13	Training 52
Drug 6	Need 71	Transfusions 4
Drugs 3	Nurse 11	Work 21
Dying 6	Nurses 96	Workshops 6
Education 4	Patients 3	
Empathy 8	People 59	
Facts 6	Person 45	
Family 4	Personal 25	
Fear 31	Prejudices 3	
Feel 10	Problems 7	
	Psychiatric 4	

Figure 6.3 : Examples of Words Used by Respondents, in Rank Order, Alphabetically (n = 21 transcripts)

Professional/ medical Words	Personal/emotional Words	Educational Words
AIDS Counselling Nurses Skills Counsellors Qualities Work Listening Nurse HIV Health Disease Empathy Specialist Drug Psychiatric Burnout Transfusions Confidentiality Disorders Drugs Patients Psychological Setting	Fear Response Need People Personal Difficult Gay Feel Death Gays Involved Problems Dying Judgemental Sexual Support Sexuality Family Caring Prejudices Help Social	Training Discussed Information Knowledge Workshop Facts Learning Groups Attitudes Education Taught
Total no of words in this category : 24 (42%)	Total no of words in this category : 22 (39%)	Total no of words in this category :11 (19%)

Figure 6.4: Words Sorted According to Categories (n = 57 words)

Category of lexical words	Total number of occurences of lexical words in transcripts (n = 57 lexical words)	Percentage of total number of lexical words identified in transcripts
Professional/ medical	736	54%
Personal/ emotional	496	36%
Educational	132	10%
Totals	1364	100%

Figure 6.5 : Frequency of Occurence of Words in the Transcripts, According to Categories (n = 1364 total occurences of words)

Category of lexical words	Total number of occurences of lexical words in transcripts (n = 56 lexical words)	Percentage of total number of lexical words identified in transcripts
Professional/ medical ('AIDS' not counted)	496	44%
Personal/ emotional	496	44%
Educational	132	12%
Totals	1124	100%

Figure 6.6 : Frequency of Occurence of Words in the Transcripts, According to Categories (n = 1124 total occurences of words), with 'AIDS' not Counted

Formal content analysis of phrases

After the content analysis of words, a formal content analysis of phrases was attempted with certain key phrases that seemed to being used frequently in the interviews. Those phrases where then extracted and an analysis of frequency of their being used throughout all of the interviews was conducted using the index feature of the wordprocessor, WordPerfect. The result of this analysis is offered in figure 6.7. The obvious limitation of this approach is that it means that only phrases used in an exact form will be identified. Thus, the phrase 'counselling skills' can be identified throughout the transcripts only if it appears in that format. The phrase 'counselling skill' will not be identified by such means.

Phrases and Number of Times Phrase Used in Transcripts
17 People with AIDS
14 Counselling skills
10 Person with AIDS
4 AIDS counsellors
4 Drug users
4 Non judgemental
4 Terence Higgins Trust
3 Why me?
3 Fear of dying
3 Self awareness
3 Safe sex
3 Legal issues
3 Sex education
3 Modes of transmission
3 Psychiatric nurses
2 Body Positive

Figure 6.7 : Examples of Phrases Used by Respondents, in Rank Order (n = 21 transcripts)

Perhaps the most notable feature of this form of analysis is that it identified that most people used the term 'person with AIDS' or 'people with AIDS' to describe the client they were talking about. This is in keeping with current trends to avoid phrases such as 'person suffering from AIDS'. Whilst there are numerous reasons for this use of language, that are well described in the literature, there is also a counter argument for its use. In ensuring that the words 'suffering' or 'victim' and similar are avoided, it is possible that the disease is somehow being sanitised in some way or even demedicalised. It is notable, for example, that it is still possible to talk of 'victims' in the context of road accidents, coronaries or even cancer. Also, the restriction of descriptors in this way is reminiscent of the 'politically correct' use of language that is being advocated in some parts of the USA. Whilst some may argue that such correctness is appropriate, some may also view it as a narrowing of the use of language and enforcing a particular and usually conservative view of the world. One of the reasons for avoiding expressions such as 'suffering from AIDS' is to avoid a particular sort of labelling. Ironically, though, many writers in the field have now abreviated the term 'people with AIDS' to "PWA's", thus adding a new label to already large number that are already available both within and without the medical profession. This remains a controversial and debatable area.

This question of a style of language has implications for the ways in which health professionals and others view the world in which they work, teach and learn and how they think about and conceptualise AIDS. Postman and Weingartner (1969) reporting on the work of Sapir and Whorf report as follows :

> [Whorf and Sapir's] studies of the language systems of different cultures led them to the conclusion...that each language - including both its structure and its lexicon represented a unique way of perceiving reality. They believed that we are imprisoned, so to speak, in a house of language. We try to assess what is outside the house from our position within it. However, the house is oddly shaped (and no one knows precisely what a normal shape would be). There is a limited number of windows. The windows are tinted and are at odd angles. We have no choice but to see what the structure of the house permits us to see. (Postman and Weingartner 1969 : 42).

Boudieu (1971) supports this application of Sapir and Whorf's work to the field of styles of language as well as to the language itself when he writes :

> What is usually known as the Sapir-Whorf hypothesis is perhaps never so satisfactorily applicable as to intellectual life; words, and especially figures of speech and figures of thought that are characteristic of a school of thought, mould thought as much as they express it. Linguistic and intellectual patterns are all the more important in determining what individuals take as worthy of being though and what they think of it in that they operate outside all critical awareness (Boudieu 1971 : 195).

And here is an important point : the language that we use to talk about AIDS may be, as it were, worked out below the level of consciousness. It is as though the language we use traps us into thinking in certain ways. This not only has implications for the work of AIDS counsellors and for traininers but also for anyone who is working in the field of AIDS education.

Content analysis of themes

This section offers the findings of the content analysis of themes. The findings that are offered here are presented as a series of tables illustrating particular perceptions, rank ordered, according to how many of the respondents mentioned the particular issue. In order to qualify for inclusion in a particular table, the responded must have mentioned the issue at least once and in context. The findings are presented under category headings. This method of analysis allowed for a much greater degree of flexibility on the part of the researcher. Rather than depending upon literal searches carried out by computer programs, the researcher was able to manual filter through the transcripts for examples of themes

Concerns of the person with AIDS

Findings, here, related to questions about what respondents felt were the main psychosocial concerns facing the person with AIDS or HIV. Sometimes this was asked as a direct question and sometimes the responses noted here were offered spontaneously by the respondents. The main responses are illustrated in figure 6.8.

Notably high, here, was the notion of stigmatisation. Many respondents referred to people with AIDS as feeling as though they were being treated as lepers and one used the term 'leperisation' to denote this process. Worry about health was clearly a concern as was fear of dying. This fear was often felt to involve families and partners. Often, respondents noted that the person with AIDS feared for the future of survivors. One respondent summed up a range of the problems that the person with AIDS can experience :

> "They are often afraid of what friends and family may think, afraid of being ill and then afraid of dying."

Perceived Psychosocial Concerns of the Person With AIDS	
Identified Concern	Number of respondents identifying this concern (n=21).
Stigmatisation	10
Worry about health	9
Fear of dying	9
Concerns about relationships	8
Financial and job worries	7
Fear of rejection	5
Anger and depression	5
Homophobia	4

Figure 6.8 : Perceived Psychosocial Concerns of the Person With AIDS or HIV

Appropriate helpers

Respondents expressed views on who they felt were best placed to help the person with AIDS or HIV with their psychosocial problems. These views are indicated in figure 6.9.

Suggested Appropriate Helpers	
Suggested Helper	Number of respondents suggesting this helper (n=21).
AIDS counsellors	7
Nurses or other health care workers	6
Partner or friend	5
AIDS organisations (Terence Higgins Trust etc)	5
Another person with AIDS	5
Buddies	2
Self-help groups	1

Figure 6.9 : Suggested Appropriate Helpers for the Person With AIDS or HIV

The most frequent response, here, was that AIDS counsellors were best placed to help the person with AIDS or HIV, followed, closely, by nurses or other health care workers (often including medical workers). Partners and friends, the voluntary organisations and other people with AIDS were all cited equally frequently. One respondent suggested that what was needed was :

> "Someone who you can be terribly personal with and can share anything with."

Buddies were only mentioned by two of the respondents and one of these suggested how difficult the tasks of being a buddy was. He suggested that the incidence of burnout in buddying was high.

AIDS and the person in the street

Respondents were asked to comment on how they felt the 'person in the street' viewed the person with AIDS or HIV. Their responses are illustrated in figure 6.10. It should be noted that what is happening here is that respondents are giving their views of what the person in the street feels about people with AIDS. Another approach to this issue would be to ask the person in the street for his or her views but that would be another study.

"Person in the Street's" View of AIDS	
Characteristic	Number of respondents who cited this characteristic (n=21).
Frightened by AIDS	11
People with AIDS are gay	9
People with AIDS deserve it	7
Ignorant of AIDS	7
Church sects may have negative views of AIDS	6
People with AIDS are being punished	4
People with AIDS are like lepers	4
People don't think about it	3

Figure 6.10 : The "Person in the Street's" View of the Person With AIDS or HIV

The most frequently used word in this context was 'fear'. Following this finding, a content analysis of words used in the interviews was conducted using a computer program that rank ordered the frequencies of all words used in a document (Carney 1982). This form of content analysis revealed that 'fear' was the noun often used throughout the combined text of the interview transcripts when making any allusion to people's feelings about AIDS.

Much homophobic prejudice was also thought to exist and a number of the respondents expressed the idea that some sects of the Church were still hostile towards people with AIDS and particular towards gay people who also had AIDS. This was expressed, by one respondent, in this way :

> "Fundamentalist sects of the church have difficulty with it. They feel it to be a moral issue and that AIDS people are sinners."

A minority thought that the average person did not think about AIDS at all. Notable, in this part of the study was the frequency with which respondents stated that they thought the person in the street associated AIDS with being gay :

> [the man in the street sees people with AIDS as] "nasty, wicked people who are all homosexual..."

> " Most of the AIDS victims in this country are perceived as being male and probably homosexuals or drug users."

A number suggested that AIDS was still seen as a 'gay plague' which is consistent with other reports on the topic (Wellings and Wadsworth 1990, Fitzpatrick and Milligan 1990).

What else needs to be done to help?

Respondents expressed views on what further work needed to be done to help people with AIDS and HIV. These are illustrated in figure 6.11.

What else needs to be done?	
Identified Need	Number of respondents identifying need (n=21).
More education about AIDS	11
Better advertising campaigns	5
More publicity about AIDS	4
More hospices and special units	4

Figure 6.11 : Perceptions of What Else Needs to be Done to Help People With AIDS and HIV

By far the most frequently suggested need was that of education of the general public. Often, this was slanted towards the need to continue education as a preventative method. Education was also seen as a requirement for changing people's attitudes towards people with AIDS and HIV and was linked to the stigmatisation, discussed above.

The government advertising campaigns were often thought to be ineffective, particularly the 'Iceberg' television campaign (Dorn and South 1990). The more direct approach of more recent advertising was appreciated but more needed to be done on the advertising front as a further means of preventing the spread of AIDS. Ironically, though, it was the 'Iceberg' series of advertisements that were most often referred to - suggesting, perhaps, that although the respondents did not feel them to be particularly effective, they were, at least, memorable!

Nurses and AIDS counselling

Few of the respondents felt that all nurses need to train as AIDS counsellors but almost all expressed the view that all nurses should have a knowledge and understanding of AIDS and HIV. Respondent's views on this topic are illustrated in figure 6.12.

Nurses and AIDS Counselling	
View Expressed	Number of respondents expressing the view (n=21)
All nurses should have knowledge and understanding of AIDS and HIV	20
Not all nurses need to train as AIDS counsellors	19
AIDS should be discussed early in nurse training	19
Nurses who work with people with AIDS should also train as AIDS counsellors	13
Psychiatric nurses could train as AIDS counsellors	5
Community nurses could train as AIDS counsellors	2

Figure 6.12 : Nurses and AIDS Counselling

Almost all respondents felt it important that the issue of AIDS was introduced early into the nursing curriculum. Once expressed surprise at the possibility of all nurses not knowing about AIDS and felt that it was an essential part of the curriculum. Views were divided as to where in the curriculum it should be discussed. Many felt that it should be explored in the first few weeks of training. Others took the view that it should be treated as any other disease and not given 'special' educational priority. Many of the respondents thought that nurses who worked directly with people with AIDS should train as counsellors and some respondents thought that psychiatric nurses might train.

Elements of an AIDS counselling course for nurses

Respondents were asked to identify what elements should make up a counselling course for nurses. A wide range of elements were identified and the main ones are illustrated in figure 6.13.

Recommended Elements of AIDS Counselling Courses for Nurses	
Element	Number of respondents recommending the element (n=21).
Up-to-date information about AIDS	16
Counselling skills	15
Discussion of sexuality	9
Self-awareness	8
Listening skills	8
Knowledge of gay and drug sub-cultures	4
Visits to special units and hospices	4
Talks from people with AIDS	4

Figure 6.13 : Recommended Elements of AIDS Counselling Courses for Nurses

Whilst there was considerable disagreement about the ideal length of a counselling course for nurses with suggestions ranging from 1 - 2 day workshops to 2 year diploma courses, most of the respondents felt that up - to - date information about AIDS was the priority in a counselling course, followed by the teaching of a range of basic counselling skills. Such skills were identified as being simple questioning techniques to those of reflection and empathy development. The AIDS counsellors in the sample were particularly adamant that the ability to empathise was a necessary quality of the AIDS counsellor. Sometimes, too, there was a sense of urgency about the process of training nurses in this field :

> "I think the emphasis should be on trying to catch as many people as you can who come into contact with people with AIDS and offer them training."

A number of respondents felt that AIDS counselling courses for nurses should involve the discussion of sexuality both from the point of view of information about different sorts of sexuality and from the point of view of nurses' exploring their own sexuality. Linked to this was the notion of self-awareness and many respondents felt that counsellors had to have sorted out their own feelings about their own sexuality if they were to be effective counsellors. One respondent identified the need for nurses to explore both their sexuality and their attitude towards dying :

> "Nurses need to understand their own sexuality and dying. We are dying all the time."

Discussion

First, it must be reiterated that this was a descriptive study. It is always dangerous to generalise from descriptions and no attempt will be made to suggest that the findings from this study are in any way representative of the thoughts and feelings of the total population of AIDS counsellors and educationalists. Many of the issues discussed by the respondents are, however, also discussed in the literature on the topic. The notion of stigmatisation, for example, is written about in some detail by (Kirkpatrick 1988) and by other commentators (Strang and Stimpson 1990).

It would seem that nurses are not only being asked to consider their own views of AIDS and of sexuality but they are being warned that they may have to face the hostility of people who do not have AIDS.

It is notable that respondents in this study did not feel that all nurses should be counsellors but that all nurses should have a thorough understanding of AIDS and related conditions. The fact that there was little agreement about how long a course on counselling should run for those nurses who did want to train as counsellors, suggests that some ambiguity about the notion of 'nurses as AIDS counsellors' may exist. However, when respondents were asked to identify themes and content for an AIDS counselling course for nurses, most were able to identify a fair number. This may, of course, be a direct reflection of their own experiences of AIDS counselling courses. It would appear that the issues of whether or not to train nurses as AIDS counsellors and of how to train them require further study.

One clear skill emerged as vital in the whole process of counselling the person with AIDS and that was the skill of listening. More than any other quality or skill, the ability to listen was discussed by most people who had had experience of counselling people with AIDS. The primacy of listening as a counselling skill is borne out by the literature on other sorts of counselling (Tschudin 1991, Burnard 1989, Heron 1990).

7 The view from the counsellors (2)

This chapter offers the findings from the second analysis of the data : an in-depth content analysis in the style of grounded theory (Glaser and Strauss 1964). During this analysis, a variety of themes emerged within each of these themes could be detected a number of sub-themes. The emergent themes were :

- Personal concerns of the person with AIDS,
- Coming to terms with AIDS,
- Appropriate helpers,
- The 'person in the streets' view of the person with AIDS,
- What else needs to be done,
- Information needed to work as an AIDS counsellor,
- Skills needed to work as an AIDS counsellor,
- The difficult aspects of AIDS counselling,
- The personal qualities of the AIDS counsellor,
- Nurses and AIDS counselling,
- Elements of an AIDS counselling course,
- The most important aspects of AIDS counselling.

Each of these themes and the sub-themes is now discussed in turn.

Personal concerns

During many of the interviews, the conversation turned to the question of what were the most difficult aspects of having AIDS. Sometimes, too, the researcher asked the direct question : 'What are some of the psychosocial problems that might face a person with AIDS?' or a variant of this question.

Worry about health

The concern about health related issues where one of the most frequently discussed issues by the respondents. Various aspects of that concern were discussed from hypochondriasis to fear of death itself. Sometimes, too, respondents talked about how clients cope with being ill. One suggested that he had known clients who

> 'Could become completely blase and live recklessly'.

This was not the general feeling, however, and most respondents felt that the people they talked to in counselling wanted clear information about the condition and what to expect :

> 'They have fear of the disease process. Fear of rejection by loved ones. Fear of not knowing what to expect and how to cope with it.'

> 'Fearful of not knowing what will happen. Not knowing what AIDS is and not taking it all in. Afraid of being ill and then afraid of dying.'

Fear of rejection

Alongside the worry about health were expressed feelings of rejection and unworthiness expressed by many clients. Some respondents felt that societal norms play a large part here in forcing the person with AIDS to feel guilty :

> 'There are lots of feelings of unworthiness : all caused by the pressures of society.'

Sometimes, though, feelings of rejection were generated by people closer to home : by families, relatives and even partners :

> 'Rejection, in a world where nobody wants them, rejection by people by family, friends, a person themselves and their partner.'

Rejection was also discussed by two nurses in the study who related their experiences of fellow health professionals demonstrating both ignorance of AIDS and negative attitudes. This was illustrated through those health professionals methods of relating to and caring for people with AIDS in a hospital setting. Both talked of ignorance of methods of prevention of the spread of AIDS and of people with AIDS being treated differently to other people in the clinical setting. One spoke of a teenage boy of whom it was suspected that he may be HIV positive being examined by doctors and nurses dressed in full theatre 'greens' and thus demonstrating both insensitivity to the patient and ignorance of AIDS itself. Both respondents identified these situations as 'rejecting' ones and said that they felt that such behaviour was not particularly atypical. They felt that many nurses and a number of medical staff lacked both knowledge and sensitivity when it came to working with people with AIDS or those who were HIV positive.

Coming to terms with AIDS

Coming to terms with the fact of AIDS was a topic discussed by almost all the respondents. One of the main concerns was the problem a person had with the initial shock of having had a positive HIV test. Some respondents felt that gay men where likely to feel guilty at hearing of the diagnosis and feel that they had brought the illness on themselves. At other times, denial was thought to operate, with blank refusal to accept the diagnosis. Sometimes, though, the diagnosis came as a relief and it was felt that the new knowledge enabled some people to plan the rest of their lives more carefully, knowing - for certain - that they had AIDS. Often, fears were focused on the person's partner or their families and, as we noted above, often on not knowing what to expect :

'They may be afraid of what friends and family may think : may see it as a disease related to homosexuality : will they think I am necessarily a homosexual? '

Who can be told?

A big question for many clients was the issue of who they could tell about being HIV positive or having AIDS. Many wondered how the person they told might react. With respect to the health professions, a number wondered about the consequences of telling doctors and nurses :

'Will I get a fair deal from doctors and nurses or will they, too, stigmatise you? Will I get depressed as a result? Are the health care staff well informed?'

This raised ethical issues of whether or not it was appropriate and 'right' to automatically tell hospital and other staff of a positive result. This issue has caused considerable debate in the researcher's own lectures on ethics with groups of student nurses. Some have felt adamant that people with AIDS must disclose to hospital staff. Others have felt equally strongly that such disclosure is a violation of personal rights to privacy. It terms of the present study, the other main area of concern about disclosure was whether or not to disclose if the client was planning on travelling abroad. Many clients felt that such disclosure would destroy possibilities of travel that would otherwise be open to them. On the other hand, other clients worried that non-disclosure might cause problems later on a trip if they happened to fall ill during a period of travel.

Coming to terms with sexuality

Sexual identity issues were often discussed. One particular issue that was raised was the fact that a number of respondents had talked to people who knew they had contracted AIDS but whose families did not know that they were gay. This sometimes lead to extreme anxiety about forced disclosure. For others, it was a 'watershed experience' and provided the reason to 'come out'. This was occasionally seen as an ironic benefit of the diagnosis.

Other clients, predictably, worried about the future of their sex lives. Some decided to become celibate whilst others worried about whether or not their partners would stay with them. For some, the fact of having AIDS seemed to further cement and already strong relationship.

Stigma

Frequent reference was made by many respondents to the idea of stigmatisation. One respondent refer to the notion of 'leperisation' or the process of becoming treated as an outcast. He suggested that this was sometimes compounded by the individual him or herself in that he or she was prone to treat him or herself as a leper. In this way the guilt that was already experience by some people with AIDS was increased. One respondent asked whether in future, people with AIDS might be institutionalised as lepers and people with mental illness had been in the past :

> 'It's rather like leprosy : are the next lot of people to be put in institutions AIDS victims? AIDS victims could be the next "lepers" ?'

In many parts of the world there have been campaigns to educate the public about AIDS, methods of prevention and about safe sex. In the Netherlands, however, it was concluded that a large scale programme to educate adolescents in this field could not necessarily be deemed successful in modifying attitudes or behaviour (Schaalma, Kok, Braeken, Schopman and Deven 1991). Perhaps this issue of stigma is intimately related to the homophobia that was also identified in the present study. It is related, also, to the rejection shown by some medical and nursing staff and discussed, above, in this chapter.

Nemesis

One reaction to the news of a positive test or of finding that you had AIDS was sometimes to feel that your past was catching up with you. A number of respondents talked of clients who felt that they had developed HIV was because of something bad they had done in the past. This was further fuelled by the apparent societal view of people with AIDS 'deserving' their condition. One respondent summed up some of these feelings, thus :

> 'The person feels guilty about what they have done to deserve it. Have I done something wrong in the past? Is it all coming back to me now? Am I too blame?'

Homophobia

One particular feature that arose during a number of interviews was the question of the sexual orientation of the counsellor. Many acknowledged that they had experienced homophobia amongst the general public. Some, however, noted another problem : that some people naturally assumed that because they were AIDS counsellors, they were gay. This was a far from straightforward issue. On a number of occasions, the respondent reported that the assumption of gayness had been made but then did not elaborate upon whether or not they were. One respondent, however, noted that he was heterosexual and not perturbed by the idea that people might think him to be gay. The issue, though, is that the respondents felt that other people might assume that AIDS counsellors were gay.

Linked to this issue was a general feeling, already discussed, that the word AIDS was firmly linked with negative connotations about gay people, in many people's minds. Much work was felt to be necessary not only in order to modify people's knowledge about AIDS but to encourage them to view gay people in a more positive light. The general publics' attitude towards gay people was generally felt to have deteriorated in the last decade, after a previous decade of greater openness and toleration of differences in sexual orientation. One respondent cited a particular example of this :

> 'Today is St Patrick's Day : in the annual New York parade, one of the cardinals of the church refused to allow gays and lesbians to march : classic example of the sort of problems that face gays.'

Financial issues

Often, the issues that were discussed by clients with the respondents in this study were practical and financial ones. Issues such as whether the client could expect to retain his or her job was a common anxiety as was the issue of whether or not a person would have problems getting a mortgage once they were found to be HIV positive or had AIDS. As a number of the respondents noted, HIV and AIDS can debar you from certain sorts of insurance. The issue became more complicated and something of an ethical dilemma when it came to disclosing whether or not you had been AIDS tested. Again, some insurance companies were thought to take a negative view of anyone who had been tested, whether or not that test subsequently proved to be positive or negative. One respondent described this as 'financial stigma'. The problems of getting insurance once you have been diagnosed as having AIDS are discussed in a number of booklets published by the Terence Higgins Trust.

Appropriate helpers

The issue of who might be the appropriate person to counsel the person with AIDS was addressed by all respondents. A comprehensive list of the people who where felt to be appropriate in helping with psychosocial problems is as follows :

- AIDS counsellors. Sometimes it was felt that these should always be trained counsellors. Others felt that there was an important place for the volunteer.
- Buddies and particularly those associated with the Terence Higgins Trust.
- Nurses. Nurses in the psychiatric field were thought to be particular useful in this area.
- Friends and partners. As one respondent suggested : 'people who love them for themselves...'.
- Other people with AIDS,
- Specialist agencies, including the London Lighthouse, Terence Higgins Trust and AIDS helplines.
- Social workers.
- Gay people. Some respondents felt it important that the gay client had access to a gay counsellor. One respondent put it like this : '[the person should be] a well trained professional who is also homosexual if the client is homosexual. Tempting to say friends but they may not want to help.'
- Self-help groups.

Some respondents felt that there was not a satisfactory counselling services so far established which really catered for the needs of people with AIDS. Others felt that it would take a long time for a person to find the right person to help them. One respondent felt that a person who was involved in AIDS counselling would have had to face their own sexuality and be clear about their own sexual needs and motives.

Person in the streets view of the person with AIDS

Another issue that was frequently discussed was the 'person in the street's' view of the person with AIDS. As was noted in the last chapter, this is the respondent's views of what the person in the street feels about the person with AIDS. Another study could be carried out which asks the person in the street. The majority of respondents who discussed this point felt it likely that the average person saw the person with AIDS as gay. Along with the implication that 'everyone who has AIDS is gay' went considerable homophobia. One respondent suggested that this was almost universal, in his experience :

'Homophobia...Just peel people's skin back and it's sitting there.'

Another respondent felt that a number of different sorts of people were often lumped together in the mind of the person in the street :

'Most of the AIDS victims in this country are perceived as being male and probably homosexuals or drug users.'

Another thought that people with AIDS might be seen by the general public as : 'Nasty, wicked people who are all homosexual or drug addicts.' Another suggested that the average person might see them as :

'Very negative. See them as diseased and like lepers. See them as very ill. Someone who has AIDS would not look 'normal'. They would be guilty and have brought it on themselves. They are being punished.'

Others felt that there was a more obvious moral dimension to many people's perception. Often it was felt by the general public that the person with AIDS deserved to have the disease or that it was their own fault and even that they did not deserve the money that was spent on them. Only one respondent felt that the person in the street's view could be positive and that was via the response : 'how can I help?'

It was often felt that fundamentalist sects of the church had difficulty with perceiving the person with AIDS in anything but a negative light. A number of respondents felt that those sects were particularly judgemental and some noted the paradox of the Christian ethic of being non-judgemental with the negative set that a number of church members held for the person with AIDS. One respondent summed up this attitude in this way :

> 'They take a religious stance. They are bigots. They say : "all AIDS sufferers are homosexual and they are being repaid for their homosexual acts.."'

Others felt that the issue of AIDS had not yet registered with the larger public. Advertising campaigns were thought to have shocked a few but made little real impact. Television advertising campaigns were picked out for special criticism. They were felt to be both unclear and uninformative. One respondent, however, felt that the situation was improving, although his response was qualified :

> 'It's getting better. People still shut their eyes unless they come into contact with a person with AIDS. Were I work, people don't think about AIDS.'

If the respondent's views really did mirror what the person in the street was thinking about the person with AIDS, it seems that the person with AIDS fears about who they tell and how they live the rest of their lives are justified. It has to be noted, however, that what is happening here is that one group of people (the respondents) are commenting on what they believe to be the perceptions of another group of people. Having said that, it seems likely that most of the respondents, given their interest in the topic, were likely to have had much to do with the 'person in the street' as well as with the person with AIDS.

What else needs to be done?

A variety of issues were discussed under the heading of 'what else needs to be done in the field of AIDS and AIDS counselling?' The most frequently discussed issue was the need for more education about AIDS. Some respondents talked about the need to further educate health care workers and seemed aware of the lack of knowledge that many health professionals had about the topic. A number highlighted the need for doctors to receive training in counselling skills.

Many respondents also discussed the need for the general public to receive more information about AIDS and safe sex through intelligent advertising campaigns. As discussed elsewhere in this book, advertising campaigns that were current at the time of data collection where felt to be totally inadequate in getting any particular message across. One respondent suggested that :

> 'There needs to be more education through effective media campaigns. Easily understandable literature which everyone can understand: cartoons and so forth. Well known people supporting the cause. Start awareness early : pre teens.'

Another issue was the need for more AIDS counselling to be made available. Some respondents felt that this should be government aided. Others felt that the counselling services that were available should be better advertised. Also, a number of respondents felt that hospital services should be improved and that more special AIDS units should be built. Others felt that special units were another way of stigmatising the person with AIDS and that present hospital facilities should be expanded to cope with the likely growth in the number of people needing care.

One respondent summed up the range of things that he felt needed to be done as follows :

> 'I would appreciate some more government led education. The television campaign was fairly poor. AIDS needs to be treated like any other illness. There are moralistic issues around. There is still an element of moralisation around. People still talk about it being a reaction to God's law.'

Information needed to work as an AIDS counsellor

Another topic discussed in the interviews was the information that a person needed in order to work as an AIDS counsellor. In keeping with much of the literature on the topic, a frequent suggestion was that an AIDS counsellor needed an up-to-date knowledge of most aspects of AIDS. The sorts of information that was discussed by respondents included the following :

- Modes of transmission,
- How to catch it and how not to catch it,
- Epidemiology,
- Infection control,
- Needle stick injuries,
- Physiology,
- Psychological effects of AIDS,
- Spiritual issues and AIDS,
- Understanding of counsellor's own sexuality,
- Legal and financial knowledge,
- Where a person can get financial advice,
- The gay sub-culture,
- The drug abuse sub-culture,
- Resources to help the person : health service, social service, voluntary.
- An understanding of one's own sexuality and one's own motives for wanting to be an AIDS counsellor.

One respondent felt that all AIDS counsellors should have access to the National AIDS Manual.

Skills needed to work as an AIDS counsellor

A variety of skills were identified as necessary in order to work as an AIDS counsellor. These were :

- Listening skills : how to listen and empathise with callers, being able to paraphrase and reflect, allowing people space to express themselves etc.
- Advice-giving skills : being able to offer clear and accurate information and advice,

- Advocacy skills : being able to stand up for the client and act on his behalf,
- A mixture of client-centred and directive counselling skills : Rogerian approaches were discussed by a number of respondents but some also discussed the need to combine client-centred counselling methods with a more confronting and prescriptive approach.

One respondent suggested that there was no difference between the skills of AIDS counselling and those of other sorts of counselling.

Difficult aspects of AIDS counselling

A number of aspects of AIDS counselling were identified as being particularly difficult. These were :

- Facing your own anxieties,
- Facing death and dying,
- Dealing with anger,
- Remaining optimistic,
- Coping with burnout,
- Telephone counselling : a particular problem.

Facing your own anxieties

This included feelings of inadequacy and of not knowing what to say. It also included the issue of how the counsellor, themselves, felt about AIDS and wondering what it must be like to experience AIDS. One respondent suggested that :

> 'Sometimes your partner or friends may not be supportive. People are nervous of the person who looks after people with AIDS'.

Another respondent expressed the almost paradoxical feelings that he had. On the one hand, he was totally committed to the process of AIDS counselling, but on the other, he was plague by doubts and uncertainties that were obviously difficult to put into words but which seemed to almost mirror some of the prejudices that 'society' expressed:

'I have no problems with people who are gay or with the AIDS issue but when it came down to it, it was just something in the back of my mind. The way that I was feeling was completely alien to the way I think normally and I felt quite guilt about it. I pride myself on being non-judgemental and yet I felt there was something wrong in the whole AIDS business...'

Another summed up some of his ambiguity about the role like this :

'You are working in an area where you are potentially being challenged about your own prejudices and sexuality.'

Facing death and dying

The AIDS counsellor always had to face the reality of the fact that at some time the client would die. Those who had been AIDS counsellors for some time found this aspect of the role the most difficult of all. One respondent put it like this :

'Having buddied two people who have died, seeing a person in the last stages before death, its a real loss, one that you ever get over. You need to have a break of about 6 months if this happens in buddying.'

Another respondent talked of the problem of helping someone who is facing a lingering death :

'You could be looking after someone for a long time who looks fairly well but suddenly registers with you that they are going to die.'

All of the respondents who had faced death in this way spoke of the need for personal preparation and for needing time for quite reflection after the client had dies. One spoke of how important it was to support the family after the client had dies. Another discussed the general fear of death and dying and the effects of death on other people :

'People's fear of death. Dealing with relatives and close friends and partners. Feelings of inability to help.Difficult to know what you can and can't do. Lack of sympathetic resources.'

Green and Sherr (1989) identify the following issues that a person who is dying may consider and which will be of practical use to counsellors in the field :

- Making a will.
- Particularly with gay couples where the partner has not got the legal status of next-of-kin (as wife or husband would have), they may need to take steps to secure the partner's financial future.
- Stating any special request of making special arrangements for the funeral. Sometimes people want special music, or a special oration. Sometimes people go even further. Several PWA's we have seen have made all their own funeral arrangements as far as possible, down to choosing the sort of coffin they want.
- Any religious requirements they may have either at the time of death, or as death approaches, or after death.
- Deciding where they want to die. Some people have a clear with to die at home if at all possible.
- Anyone they would want to be with them when they are dying.
- Who should be informed when they are dying.
- Putting personal papers together and leaving any special instructions about their affairs (Green and Sherr 1989).

The issue of the counsellor having to cope with his or her own feelings about death and dying are highlighted by Goldblum and Moulton :

> Clinicians must face their own death anxiety. Uncertainty regarding the course of the illness [AIDS] may be unsettling to clinicians as well as to clients. (Goldblum and Moulton 1989).

It would seem that part of the business of helping the client to face his or her death is also the process of working through your own fear of dying.

Dealing with anger

A number of respondents talked of the problem of coping with client's anger. Often, this anger was projected onto the counsellor. One respondent talked of how difficult it was to be rejected by the client : 'What do you do when the person tells you to bugger off?' Dealing with overt anger and aggression was sometimes frightening and many of the respondents felt that these issues needed to be discussed in AIDS counselling training courses. Methods for helping people express their feelings were described in a previous chapter. As Heron (1977) notes, however, facing anger is perhaps the most difficult in a counselling or group setting in that it is not only personally threatening but potentially physically threatening too. Acevedo has this to say about the issue of anger and of the need to set boundaries :

> Angry feelings need to be acknowledged and accepted. While anger is a natural and common reaction to situations like AIDS that makes us feel powerless, it is not acceptable to threaten individuals or the group, and strong limit setting may be necessary (Acevedo 1989.

Remaining optimistic

Just as the client would often find it difficult to remain cheerful or purposeful, so, too, did the respondents. One, reflecting on the possibility of becoming a counsellor, suggested that :

> 'I would find it hard to be optimistic and positive when the outcome is so severe.'

Another, an active counsellor, talked of the difficulty of keeping going in counselling :

> 'All you can do is try to alleviate some of suffering. You can't take it away. There is no cure.'

The question of optimism and hope is an important one. Perhaps the most stressful situation of all is the fact of having an inability to find meaning at all. Such a state may be described as dispiritedness . Dispiritedness, then, is the fact of being unable to invest life with meaning. It is sometimes, but not always, combined with depression. When it is not, it is characterised by a general sense of loss, a lack of conviction in what one is doing and a lack of enthusiasm for life in general. It may also be accompanied by a sense of cynicism and by the development of 'gallows humour'.

Some commentators have gone further and formally defined the notion of spiritual distress. Kim, McFarland, and McLane (1987) define spiritual distress as

> 'distress of the human spirit...a disruption in the life principle which pervades a person's entire being and which integrates and transcends one's biological and psychosocial nature.'

It may be argued, in passing, that the first part of this definition is tautological and that the second raises questions about what we are to understand by the idea of 'the life principle'. Kim, McFarland and McLane go on to offer defining characteristics of spiritual distress. These are :

- Expresses concern with meaning of life/death or any belief system,
- Anger towards God,
- Questions meaning of suffering,
- Verbalises inner conflict about beliefs,
- Verbalises concern about relationships with deity,
- Questions meaning of own existence,
- Unable to participate in usual religious practices,
- Seeks spiritual assistance,
- Questions moral or ethical implications of therapeutic regimen,
- Gallows humour,
- Displacement of anger toward religious representatives
- Nightmares of sleep disturbance,
- Alteration of behaviour or mood evidenced by anger, crying, withdrawal, preoccupation, anxiety, hostility or apathy (Kim, McFarland and McLane 1987).

This notion of spiritual distress appears to suggest that it is something that may occur in those who have previously held religious beliefs and who are now questioning them. It is suggested here that the notion of spiritual distress may be better conceptualised as a concern with ultimate things and with meaning. In this way, it is quite possible to argue that atheists and agnostics are just as capable of experiencing spiritual distress as are those who have, or who have had, religious convictions (Burnard 1988). Spiritual distress, in these terms, is characterised more than anything else by a profound sense of meaninglessness.

In the case of the person who has AIDS, the meaningless may come from a questioning of why one has caught AIDS - the 'why me?' question. This question was one that was frequently identified by AIDS counsellors and others as one that people with AIDS tended to ask themselves and it was often linked to the notion of nemesis, discussed in this chapter. Macks, discussing the question of hope in the context of AIDS, writes as follows :

> Maintaining hope is a primary task for every person with AIDS, and it is one of the most difficult. Feelings of hope fluctuate daily, and sources of hope differ from person to person. Maintaining hope is a daily process, not a state that is ultimately attained. The degree of hope people feel can be affected drastically by how well they feel physically, emotionally or spiritually that day. Hope is fostered when individuals feel powerful and in control of their lives to as great a degree as possible (Macks 1989).

Burnout

Related to the issues of death and dying and to the issue of remaining optimistic was that of burnout. Burnout is the sensation of profound emotional exhaustion caused by job-related stress (Burnard 1990). One respondent described the problem thus :

> 'Working from long periods with client: that can be tiring on the counsellor and difficult for the person with AIDS and get dependent. Sometimes it all seems to get too much and I think I'm going to pack it in.'

Sometimes, the problem was one of lack of support. The following respondent not only talked of the difficulty of taking your work home with you but also of finding someone with whom you could discuss your own fears and anxieties as an AIDS counsellor. He seems to suggest, too, that you may be stigmatised by association :

> 'If your counselling someone with cancer you take your work home but with HIV you may not feel that you can discuss it with others. Sometimes your partner or friends MAY NOT be supportive. People are nervous of the person who looks after people with AIDS. You need to allow people to air their anxieties.'

Sometimes, burnout was a result of not being appreciated as a counsellor. In many ways, there seemed to be few direct rewards for being an AIDS counsellor, beyond the intrinsic reward of being motivated to help others : 'Our work is not being seen as important : we are not valued.'

At other times, the personal involvement with the client led to exhaustion and a feeling of burnout :

> 'It's a problem : the inner quality, the ability to stay calm. They have to be prepared to allow themselves to get fairly close to the person. For example the heterosexual person working with the gay person : it all causes a lot of conflicts. One problem in the AIDS counselling field is that people may bring in their own problems and this may be a problem. I don't bring my own sexuality into my work : you can't.'

The term burnout is usually used to describe the feelings associated with long-term, job related stress. Maslach suggests that:

> Burnout is a syndrome of emotional exhaustion, depersonalization, and reduced personal accomplishment that can occur among individuals who do 'people work' of some kind. It is a response to the chronic emotional strain of dealing extensively with other human beings, particularly when they are troubled or having problems. Thus, it can be considered one type of job stress. (Maslach 1981).

Burnout is usually associated with working in caring professions, under considerable stress, for long periods. Characteristics include:

- loss of motivation,
- the development of negative rather than positive attitudes towards the job and towards other people,

- the development of a 'gallows' sense of humour or a loss of sense of humour altogether,
- a sense of a narrowing choice of options,
- a feeling that one is acted upon rather than exercising choice.

Maslach (1981) identifies three stages in the process of burnout : 1) emotional exhaustion, 2) depersonalisation and 3) feelings of reduced personal accomplishment.

Emotional exhaustion

The first characteristic of the onset of burnout is a sense of emotional fatigue. The carer feels that she has little left to give to others and begins to cope with this by gradually cutting herself off from others. This leads to stage two, the stage of depersonalisation.

Depersonalisation

In this stage, the fact of cutting oneself off from others as a coping strategy leads to a sense of alienation from others. Others are also viewed in a negative light and the health professional often begins to actively dislike those people that she previously cared for or worked with. It is not uncommon to hear health professionals remark in a cynical way 'this job would be O.K. if it weren't for the clients'... for the person experiencing burnout, this sentiment becomes a reality. Often the person expends a lot of energy in trying to avoid clients and other people. Sometimes this is through burying herself in paperwork and administration. Sometimes it is by keeping appointments very brief. Overall, the feeling is one negative attitudes towards self and others.

Reduced personal accomplishment

All of this distancing takes its toll. The person experiencing burnout ends up by feeling that they are achieving very little. In some cases this is true. In others, the negative attitudes lead to an inability to self-assess and to evaluate work outcomes. Sometimes, all past work is 'rubbished'. The burnout person comes to feel that nothing she has done in the field of caring has been worthwhile and that if she had previously viewed herself as caring, she had been deluded. It is at this point that many people choose to leave the profession all together and seek work in a situation where they can avoid others. Others learn to cope by adopting a distant or cynical approach towards other people.

Coping with burnout

Pines, Aronson and Kafry (1981) suggest three major strategies for coping with burnout:

- being aware of the problem,
- taking responsibility for doing something about it,
- achieving some degree of cognitive clarity,
- developing new tools for coping.

Being aware of the problem

The first stage must be recognising that a problem exists at all. This is not always easy as the process of burnout is often so insidious. Sometimes the change of attitude in the person experiencing burnout is noted by a colleague and this offers the chance for discussion of the problem. Even then, it is common for the burntout person to deny that anything is wrong or if there is, to see the problem as being external to themselves. Very often, that person's distress is displaced onto the job, the organisation or onto other people. Thus it is not uncommon to hear people suffering from this type of stress reaction to claim that the organisation 'no longer cares' for them, or that 'the job has changed and isn't interesting any more'. Rarely can the person 'own' the problem and identify that whilst the job and the clients have contributed to burnout, the problem lies within. This recognition must occur if something is to change.

Taking responsibility for doing something about it

Linked to identifying that a problem exists is the recognition that if anything is to change, the person with burnout must take the initiative in doing something about it. Unfortunately, this is usually what they feel least able to do. They often feel powerless and demotivated to the point of merely being able to struggle through. This is where help from other colleagues and friends can make the difference. Through talking through the issues and through being heard by another person, the carer with burnout can come to the decision to change her situation.

Achieving cognitive clarity

Burnout has a distinct emotional component. As we have noted, the burntout person often feels trapped and disinterested. The point, in this stage, is to carefully itemise exactly what the issues are that are contributing to the state of burnout. It is never only the case that a person feels emotionally exhausted. Things are happening to them that make them feel that way. Through careful analysis of what is happening in the person's life and in their work can lead to the identification of solutions.

Developing new skills for coping

The process of gaining cognitive clarity leads to the development of ways of coping with burnout. Nothing else changes unless a behavioural change occurs. The first stage in achieving such behavioural change is the identification of clear objectives, as noted above. This is not to suggest that everything that contributes to a person feeling burnout can be changed but to suggest that with clear goals, some things can be changed. The point about such goals is that they need to be clearly stated and achievable.

Telephone counselling : a particular problem

Telephone counselling was seen by some respondents as different to other sorts. For one respondent, the problem was sometimes deciding on the genuineness of the caller : he summed this up with a general preface about his perception of the difficult part of AIDS counselling :

'For those of us who haven't got AIDS its difficult to empathise with the horror of it. Also, the hoax caller is difficult. The thought sometimes occurs to you : " am I being strung along here?".'

Personal qualities of an AIDS counsellor

A number of specific personal qualities for the AIDS counsellor were refereed to by respondents. These were as follows and echo the personal qualities described in the literature and in an earlier chapter of this book :

- Being non-judgemental
- Being positive,
- Being involved and committed,
- Understanding,
- Unconditional love,
- Being accepting,
- Empathic,
- Warm.

These qualities discussed by the respondents in the study also strongly echo those recommended by Rogers (1967) as necessary and sufficient qualities for therapeutic change. One respondent spelt out what he felt to be the particular personal qualities of an effective counsellor and seems to be calling for a secure and 'safe' person :

'Those that have some sort of psychiatric nursing would, in theory, be better than general nurses. It depends more on the character of the person. A nice plump middle aged person might be better than a slightly neurotic, intense young person with a degree.'

Nurses and AIDS counselling

Few respondents felt that all nurses should train as AIDS counsellors but all felt that nurses should have a full understanding of AIDS and the consequences of having AIDS. Some felt that the problem of AIDS was small enough for a handful of nurses to be trained as AIDS counsellors. Others felt that particular sorts of nurses should be trained including psychiatric nurses, childrens nurses and those who were likely to look after people with AIDS. One felt that training nurse as AIDS counsellors would be a waste of money and that such training should be reserved for people who had a special interest in it. Some were specific about the sorts of nurses and the sorts of training that should be offered :

> 'We are looking for really good counsellors so they should have a degree or diploma in counselling, perhaps through open learning. That could be being achieved whilst they are working in the AIDS setting.'

By far the most frequent response in this area was that all nurses should have an understanding of AIDS and all aspects of AIDS. Examples of responses of this sort included :

> 'All nurses should have a good knowledge of AIDS and should be taught to cope with things that arise. Also to keep themselves safe.'

> 'Probably all nurses should have some knowledge of the subject. The right sort of nurses can be trained in counselling as is true of social workers or psychologists.'

Some respondents felt that the AIDS question should be 'normalised' and that AIDS should not be treated as a special case. An example of this sort of response is as follows :

> 'It ought to be discussed as a general illness. We need to get to the stage were it is treated as just another illness.'

Others felt that nurses need to consider their own sexuality in the light of AIDS and AIDS counselling. It was one thing to teach people to listen and to counsel but another to get nurses to accept the person who is HIV positive or who has AIDS. The sexuality issue was discussed by a number of respondents :

> 'Nurses need to think about what to do if they are being turned on by the person with AIDS or how to face their feelings. Great

need to know how to touch another person. You need to be safe in your own sexuality.'

'Nurses need to know enough to know how to approach the person with AIDS. They need to understand their own sexuality and dying.'

Another, discussing the need for nurses to have explored their sexuality and their knowledge bases about AIDS and HIV, found it : 'quite frightening to think that nurses might not know much about AIDS.' Perhaps a general view, held by the general public, might be that nurses did know about AIDS. The respondents in this study seemed to feel that nurses did not know enough. A number also felt that this was true of doctors and the medical profession.

'There is a need for educating the health care worker right across the board. Doctors in particular, there is a real need for counselling skills for doctors. Everybody needs education.'

Elements of an AIDS counselling course

A variety of views were expressed about what should go into the design of an AIDS counselling course. These can be identified as follows :

- **Up to date knowledge of all aspects of AIDS** : Information about AIDS, Safe sex, Contraception, Basic counselling techniques and theory, Development of AIDS and history. Causes.Information element on AIDS itself. Life sciences element. Psychosocial elements Spiritual, emotional side of it. History of AIDS. Differing views of it. The statistical side of it. Making trainees realise that it is not a 'Gay Plague'. Information about (up to date) about AIDS. Social consequences, Financial consequences, Psychological consequences.

- **Counselling skills and listening skills,**
- **Sexuality : homosexuality/heterosexuality**
- **The experience of having AIDS** : Visits to centres who help people with AIDS and special clinics. Talks from people like the TH Trust and other organisations. Meeting people with full blown AIDS. People from self-help groups. The nitty gritty of how the disease is

caught. Examination of attitudes : why do you want to be an AIDS counsellor? Who should be AIDS counsellors? Have people with AIDS talk to them. Have someone who is really ill to see the trainees.

Also, ethical questions were deemed important as part of the curriculum. During the course of the interviews, some respondent's identified their own ethical positions. One had particularly strong views on this issue and felt that :

> 'I know it's very controversial but I would like mandatory testing which would promote the common good and which would bring the least cost to the individual. I regret that it has not been made a notifiable disease. I think everyone should be tested when they come into hospital.'

Conclusion

A wide range of issues were discussed by the respondents in this study and any report has to be selective : not all themes from all interviews could be presented in a report like this. This is one of the problems of reporting qualitative studies. In one sense, the only real way to do justice to what people say in a study of this sort would be to present the full transcripts of the interviews, bound and in book form. On the other hand, the researcher must seek for patterns and must make some decisions about inclusion and exclusion whilst seeking to represent what people have said fairly and honestly.

Some themes were recurring. What was clear, though, and something that cannot be demonstrated through the quotations in this analysis was the obvious commitment to the task of counselling that came through in the interviews by those who were working in that role. It would seem that although a number of problem areas are raised, the overall feeling was that AIDS counselling was satisfying work.

The issues that seem to be discussed with frequency throughout the study can be summarised thus :

- AIDS counselling calls for a range of personal qualities and strengths and causes the counsellor to reflect on his or her own beliefs, prejudices and sexual values,

- Fear is a frequently discussed emotion in AIDS counselling and yet the emotional aspect of counselling seems often to be countered more by information giving than by the exploration of personal fears.
- AIDS counselling combines elements of the non-directive, Rogerian (or client-centred) approach with a more prescriptive, advice giving approach although the prescriptive style seems to predominate,
- AIDS counsellors need an up-to-date knowledge of a wide range of aspects of AIDS and HIV related issues. Indeed the knowledge and information aspect of AIDS counselling emerges as one of its most important features,
- AIDS counsellors address a range of emotional issues in their work related both to their clients and to themselves,
- AIDS counsellors would seem to need support from others (perhaps in the form of support groups) and often feel vulnerable and sometimes undervalued.
- Not all nurses need to train as AIDS counsellors but all nurses should have a broad and deep understanding of AIDS and AIDS related conditions.

It is not possible to generalise nor extrapolate from descriptive studies of this sort but the study does appear to support some of the findings of other researchers and writers in the field. Perhaps the most notable finding is the one that reinforces the need for up-to-date information on the part of the AIDS counsellor. Many writers on the question of AIDS counselling have discussed the educative aspect of the work (Green and McCreaner 1989, Dilley, Pies and Helquist 1989, Bor 1991, Bor, Miller, Perry et al 1991) and this must be a central focus of the work (although this point is discussed again, later in this chapter). What the AIDS worker always has to face is the fact that, as yet, there is no sign of a cure for AIDS and that all medical intervention is likely to be of a palliative nature. This will, in turn, produce all sorts of emotional sequelae that will have to be addressed by the AIDS counsellor. That counsellor is working in a position that is not often valued by other members of society and yet he or she constantly faces the task of offering emotional support to other people. Another important issue that arises out of this study is the need for support for the counsellors. Finally, it would appear that AIDS counselling blends two sorts of approaches to counselling : the client-centred and the prescriptive. It is one thing to offer clear and unambiguous information, it is another to cope with the effects of that information and with the results of suffering from a disease for which no cure is known. Figure 7.1. identifies some of the differences and similarities between AIDS counselling and other sorts of counselling, drawing from both the findings of this study and from the literature on the topic. Notable points in this comparison are the relatively short history of AIDS counselling : it may be anticipated that AIDS counselling will develop and grow in many and different ways over the next few years; the medical bias of a lot of AIDS counselling. Also, as we have seen throughout this study, AIDS counselling has tended to be more prescriptive and informative than other sorts of counselling. This was summed up by one respondent in the study, who worked on an AIDS helpline, as follows :

> 'A lot of the counselling that is done is still on questions of practical information : little seems to be being done on some of the emotional concerns of people with AIDS.'

In the next chapter, a framework is offered for combining both the facilitative and the prescriptive aspects of the work.

These, then, are some of the differences between AIDS counselling and more traditional approaches to counselling. An important question arises out of the findings of this study and out of the literature on the topic of AIDS counselling. It is this : does the providing of clear information on a particular topic change behaviour? If AIDS counselling is concerned to a considerable degree with the provision of up-to-date information, then it may be imagined that one of the reasons such information is given is that it will help to change the behaviour of the people to whom that information is given. The giving of information must be predicated on the idea that people will act on the information given. However, it is far from evident that people do automatically change their behaviour as a result of being given information.

	AIDS COUNSELLING	OTHER COUNSELLING
Aim	Helping the person to come to terms with one or more aspect of AIDS	Helping the person with a variety of problems in living
Clientele	Worried well People pre-test People post-test People with AIDS Partners and families	Anyone who seeks out counselling
Counsellor	AIDS counsellor Medical practitioner Health care professional Helpline volunteer	Trained counsellor Voluntary worker Health care professional
Most frequent style of counselling	Prescriptive Informative Client-centred	Client-centred
Timespan of counselling relationships	Short term OR Until client terminates relationships or client dies	Open ended : often lengthy
Theoretical base	Often medical	Often psychological Often humanistic or psychodynamic
History of counselling	From 1981	From early 20th century

Figure 7.1 : Comparison of AIDS Counselling and Other Counselling

With regard to sex education, it has been suggested that only when sex education is explicitly tailored to the behaviours in question is it likely to produce a behavioural change (Kirby 1985, Kok 1990). In order to produce behavioural changes, it would appear that educational programmes should include cognitive and behavioural skills training addressed at interpersonal problem solving and assertive communication as well as information (Gilchrist and Schinke 1983, Bandura 1983). Following an evaluation of an educational programme for adolescents in Holland about AIDS, Schaalma, Kolk, Braeken et al (1991) were uncertain about the degree to which that programme could claim to have an effect on behaviour. Also, it is interesting to note that Carl Rogers, founder of the client-centred approach, began his career by offering information as a form of therapy (Kirschenbaum 1979). He believed in the value of giving information as a means of enabling clients to make decisions about their life problems. However, Kirschenbaum notes that Rogers' :

> ...experience also taught him the limitations of the educational approach. Deep-seated emotional problems would scarcely be touched by education. *And even when ignorance of basic facts was an important part of the problem, emotional conflicts often interfered with the individual's ability to accept the facts* [emphasis added] (Kirschenbaum 1979).

It has to be said, of course, that Rogers was not dealing with AIDS. It seems possible, though, that counsellor's may need to consider more than information giving - even when the topic is so central a one as AIDS - if people's behaviour is to change or even if they are to listen to and accept that information. On this issue of behaviour and attitudes being changed as a result of information given, Aronson (1980) summarises, from the social psychology research and literature, the following issues that are salient :

- Our opinions are influenced by individuals who are both expert and trustworthy,
- A communicator's trustworthiness (and effectiveness) can be increased if he or she argues a position apparently opposed to his or her self-interest,
- A communicator's trustworthiness (and effectiveness) can be increased if he or she does not seem to be trying to influence our opinion,
- At least where trivial opinions and behaviours are concerned, if we like and can identify with a person, his or her opinions and

behaviours will be more influential upon our own that their content would ordinarily warrant,

- Again, where trivial opinions and behaviours are concerned, if we like a person, we will tend to be influenced even if it is clear that he or she is trying to influence us and stands to profit by doing so. (Aronson 1980).

All of these issues have implications for the ways in which AIDS counselling is conducted and for how AIDS prevention and education programmes are organised. It may be one thing to give people information but quite another to change their opinions or behaviour - especially on important issues. We cannot assume that giving people information in order that they can make informed decisions necessarily means that they will make informed decisions.

Summary

Figure 7.2. offers a summary of some of the issue discussed in the interviews in this study and draws out some of the salient features. Figure 7.3. develops, tentatively, a model of AIDS counselling drawn from the data.

Type of language used	Medical Personal Educational
Type of issues discussed regarding people with AIDS	Stigma Fear Death and dying Fear of rejection Financial worries Who can they tell? Partners, families, friends Homophobia etc.
Anxieties of those who counsel or who may counsel	Remaining optimistic Facing death and dying Burnout
Person in the streets view of the person with AIDS	Homosexual Drug abusers Morally judged
What else needs to be done	More information More education Specialist units
Personal qualities of the AIDS counsellor	Warmth Non-judgmental attitude Understanding Unconditional love Empathy
Training components of an AIDS counselling course	Information about AIDS Counselling skills Review of sexuality
Nurses role in AIDS counselling	Not necessarily counsellors but all should have knowledge and information about AIDS

Fig 7.2 : Summary of Some of the Issues Discussed by the Respondents

<table>
<tr><td>MEDICAL ISSUES</td><td>EDUCATIONAL ISSUES</td><td rowspan="3">Counselling Style :
Informative,
Prescriptive</td></tr>
<tr><td>Dealt with through information</td><td>Dealt with through information</td></tr>
<tr><td>Expert is in control</td><td>Expert is in control</td></tr>
<tr><td colspan="2">PERSONAL ISSUES</td><td rowspan="3">Counselling Style :
Facilitative</td></tr>
<tr><td colspan="2">Dealt with through personal involvement</td></tr>
<tr><td colspan="2">Expert and client meet on an equal footing</td></tr>
</table>

Fig 7.3 : Tentative Model of Aspects of AIDS Counselling

It may be useful to review some of the predominant issues that were discussed by the respondents in this study and to develop a tentative theory of AIDS counselling in the light of some of those responses. From the content analysis of words and from the more detailed qualitative analyses, it would appear that three domains were discussed : medical issues, personal issues and educational issues. The medical and educational aspects of the AIDS counsellor's role may help the counsellor to stay detached and in control of what is potentially an overwhelming situation. To venture into the domain of person issues is to risk all of the negative things identified by the respondents : burnout, loss of optimism and so forth. Perhaps, then, the medical and educational positions are the safer ones for the counsellor and using them may be a defensive manoeuvre, for some, in a field where there is potential for 'running out of answers'. The personal issues call for much greater personal involvement and for personal inner resources. To this end, the styles of counselling may be different in the various domains. The medical and educational issues seem to call for an informative and prescriptive style whilst the personal issues may call for a more facilitative style. These two styles are discussed in greater detail in the next chapter.

8 A model for AIDS counselling

The bases of effective AIDS counselling are the skills of listening and giving attention. Second to these comes the need to use effective verbal interventions involving both client-centred AND more prescriptive counselling. A format for understanding the range of useful and therapeutic interventions has been devised by John Heron (Heron 1986) and is called Six Category Intervention Analysis which combines both elements and may be a useful framework for planning workshops for AIDS counsellors.

This conceptual framework known was developed by Heron out of the work of Blake and Mouton (1976). It was offered as a conceptual model for understanding interpersonal relationships, and as an assessment tool for identifying a range of possible therapeutic interactions between two people.

The six categories in Heron's analysis are : prescriptive (offering advice), informative (offering information), confronting (challenging), cathartic (enabling the expression of pent-up emotions), catalytic ('drawing out') and supportive (confirming or encouraging) . The word 'intervention' is used to describe any statement that the practitioner may use. The word 'category' is used to denote a range of related interventions.

Heron (1986) calls the first three categories of intervention, (prescriptive, informative and confronting),'authoritative' and suggests that in using these categories the practitioner retains control over the relationship. He calls the second three categories of intervention (cathartic, catalytic and supportive), 'facilitative' and suggests that these enable the client to retain control over the relationship. In other words, the first three are 'practitioner-centred' and the second three are 'client-centred'. Another way of describing the difference between the first and second sets of three categories is that the first three are 'You tell me' interventions and the second three are 'I tell you' interventions.

What, then, is the value of such an analysis of therapeutic interventions? First. it identifies the range of possible interventions available to the nurse/counsellor. Very often, in day to day interactions with others, we stick to repetitive forms of conversation and response simply because we are not aware that other options are available to us. This analysis identifies an exhaustive range of types of human interventions. Second, by identifying the sorts of interventions we can use, we can act more precisely and with a greater sense of intention. The counsellor/client relationship thus becomes more particular and less haphazard : we know what we are saying and also how we are saying it. We have greater interpersonal choice.

Third, the analysis offers an instrument for training. Once the categories have been identified, they can be used for students and others to identify their weaknesses and strengths across the interpersonal spectrum Counsellors can, in this way, develop a wide range and comprehensive range of interpersonal skills.

It is worth repeating that the skills identified in this chapter as counselling skills are exactly similar to the basic human skills used in day to day nursing interactions. Thus an understanding of the full range of the six categories can enhance and enrich the quality of the counsellor's approach to care. It should be noted, too, that the analysis does not offer a mechanical approach to interpersonal skills training. The exercises here will not simply be a training in learning particular phrases and reposes. This is an important issue. The analysis indicates a type or response. The choice of words, the tone of voice, the non-verbal aspects of a particular response must develop out of the individual's belief and value system and out of their life experience. Those aspects of the response are also dependent upon the situation at the time and upon the people involved. All human relationships occur within a particular context. It is impossible to identify what will necessarily be the right thing to do in this situation at this time. A mechanical, learning-by-heart approach to counselling or interpersonal skills would, therefore, be inappropriate. In the descriptions of the following exercises, examples are offered but when the exercises are carried out, each student will have to find his own words, his own expressions and his own personal approach. This affirms the basic principle of human skills training : the honouring of personal experience developed through observation and reflection.

Nurses' perceptions of their interpersonal skills

In two recent studies, we invited both student nurses and trained nursing staff to identify their own strengths and weaknesses in terms of the Six Category Intervention Analysis (Burnard and Morrison 1988, Morrison and Burnard 1991). In the first study, using an accidental sample of 92 trained nurses, those nurses were asked to rank order the six categories according how skilful they thought they were in using them. Generally speaking the nurses perceived themselves to be more skilled in using the authoritative categories and less skilled in using the facilitative categories. Having said that, most of the nurses perceived themselves as being particularly weak in using cathartic and catalytic interventions. Overall, they perceived themselves as being best at being supportive.

There were marked similarities in the findings of the second study in which we invited 84 student nurses to rank order the six categories in terms of their perceived strengths and weaknesses in using them. Again we found an overall picture of greater perceived skill in using authoritative interventions rather than facilitative ones. Students also thought that they were generally most effective in using supportive interventions and not so good at using cathartic and confronting interventions. In general, the results of both studies support Heron's (1986) assertion that a wide range of practitioners in our society show a much greater deficit in the skilful use of facilitative interventions that they do in the skilful use of authoritative ones.

Six category intervention analysis and AIDS counselling

The intervention analysis, as we have noted, claims to be exhaustive of all possible therapeutic interventions. The analysis divides therapeutic interventions into two sorts :

- authoritative interventions
- facilitative interventions.

Drawing from the information and views offered by the respondents in this study, it is possible to identify that both sorts of interventions are required for effective AIDS counselling. AIDS counselling calls for more than just the client-centred approach and also requires that the effective counsellor is able to give appropriate advice, information and confrontation. The following diagram illustrates the sorts of ways in which the intervention analysis might act as a framework for both practising and teaching AIDS counselling.

AUTHORITATIVE INTERVENTIONS	
Prescriptive	Giving clear advice about testing. Recommending changes in sexual practice.
Informative	Offering information about AIDS, safe sex etc. Educating and training.
Confronting	Challenging current sexual activity where this is appropriate.
FACILITATIVE INTERVENTIONS	
Cathartic	Helping with feelings. Helping the person to come to terms with the experience of AIDS.
Catalytic	Drawing the client out in order to talk more about their worries, their sexual practices, their future plans.
Supportive	Supporting the client against stigmatisation and prejudice. Standing by the client throughout the experience of having AIDS.

Figure 8.1: Examples of the Application of Six Category Intervention Analysis to AIDS Counselling

Aspects of AIDS counselling training

Drawing from the literature and from the findings of this study, it is possible to identify some of the aspects that need to be considered in AIDS counselling training both for nurses and for other health professionals and volunteers. Figure 8.2. identifies some of the content of such courses and figure 8.3. some of the teaching and learning methods. The later are drawn from the literature on adult learning methods, experiential learning and interpersonal skills training methods (Knowles 1978, Jarvis, 1984, Burnard 1989, 1990, 1991).

Information	e.g. : natural history, incidence, nature, safe sex ethics, etc.
Psychosocial elements	e.g. Fear and anxiety, living with AIDS, death and dying etc.
Counselling skills	e.g. Listening and attending, questioning, reflecting, checking for understanding etc.
Support systems	e.g. Co-counselling, peer support groups, follow up study days etc.

Figure 8.2 : Content Issues for an AIDS Counselling Course

• Lectures
• Talks from people with AIDS and from other counsellors
• Talks from people from specialist agencies (e.g. Terence Higgins Trust, London Lighthouse etc).
• Discussion groups
• Experiential learning activities (e.g. pairs work, role play, structured group activities, brainstorming sessions, psychodrama etc.)
• Plenary sessions
• Self and peer evaluation
• Regular up-date sessions and follow up study days

Figure 8.3: Teaching and Learning Methods for AIDS Counselling Training

From these figures and combinations of content and methods, it is possible to identify the key elements of a training course for AIDS counselling. The following is a tentative programme of educational and training elements in the order that they may be used in a training workshop. Decisions would have to be made about how long such a training programme might be and whether it would be run as a one or two day workshop, a one or two week workshop or a series of evening or day study workshops. McCreaner (1989c) recommends the consideration of four course models :

- hourly sessions,
- specialist seminars,
- experiential workshops,
- follow up courses (McCreaner 1989c).

The nuts and bolts of organising and facilitating counselling skills and interpersonal skills workshops have been discussed in detail elsewhere (Burnard 1989). What follows is the ordering of the material to be covered in a typical workshop.

1. Welcome, icebreakers and introductions

2. Introductory lectures on AIDS and AIDS related issues
- History,
- Modes of transmission,
- Epidemiology,
- Treatments,
- Psychological, sociological and spiritual elements.

3. Discussion of the experience of AIDS
- Typical problems,
- visits from people with AIDS,
- Visits to specialist agencies,
- Values clarification,
- Sexuality

4. Introduction to counselling
- definitions,
- the counselling relationship,
- what counselling is and what it is not,
- personal qualities of the AIDS counsellor,
- Maps of the counselling relationship.

5. Introduction to Six Category Intervention Analysis
- A description of the analysis,
- Prescriptive interventions,
- Informative interventions,
- Confronting interventions,
- Cathartic interventions,
- Confronting interventions.

6. Experiential exercises in the six categories using :
- Pairs exercises,
- Role play,
- Psychodrama,
- Structured group exercises,
- Brainstorming sessions,
- Plenary group discussions.

7. Discussion of particular issues in AIDS counselling, e.g. :
- disclosing diagnosis,
- facing death and dying,
- dealing with stigmatisation,
- counsellor support,
- coping with stress and burnout,
- working on the telephone etc.

8. Evaluation of the workshop and forward planning.

Experiential learning

The term experiential learning has been used frequently in this chapter. In this section, the concept is briefly described. Clearly, people have always learned from experience. However, the idea of experiential learning as an educational concept is a relatively recent one. It will be useful to review some of the historical roots of the concept in order to make sense of some of the experiential learning methods that have been alluded to in this study.

Drawing on the work of American pragmatic philosopher, John Dewey (1916, 1938), Keeton and Associates (1976) describe experiential learning as including learning through the process of living and include work experience, skills developed through hobbies and interests and non-formal educational activities. This approach to definition is reflected in the F.E.U. project report 'Curriculum opportunity' which asserts that, for the purposes of that report, experiential learning referred to the knowledge and skills acquired through life and work experience and study (F.E.U. : 1983). Clearly, all of this is relevant to the teaching and learning of AIDS counselling. The person who has had personal experience of working with people with AIDS and who has a genuine interest in the field seems likely to be able to bring considerable experience to workshops on AIDS counselling.

Pfeiffer and Goodstein (1982) offer a different approach to the concept by describing an 'experiential learning cycle' which spells out the possible process of experiential learning (Fig 8.4) This cycle not only suggests the format for organising experiential learning but also makes tacit reference to the way in which people learn through experience.

Kolb (1984) was more explicit about this learning process in his 'experiential learning model' (Fig 8.5). In this model, concrete experience is the starting point for a reflective process that echoes Paulo Freire's (1972) concept of 'praxis'. Praxis, for Freire is the combination of reflection-and-action-on-the-world : a transforming process that is one of man's distinguishing features and one that enables him to change his view of the world and ultimately, to change the world itself. In the context of AIDS, the very fact of having AIDS or of becoming aware of it can have a transforming action on the life of the person who gains that knowledge or awareness.

1. Experiencing
2. Publishing
3. Processing (discussion of patterns and dynamics)
4. Generalising (Inferring principles about the 'real world')
5. Applying (Planning more effective behaviour)

Figure 8.4: An Experiential Learning Cycle (after Pfeiffer and Goodstein)

1. Concrete Experience
2. Observations and reflections
3. Formation of abstract concepts and generalisations.
4. Testing implications of concepts in new situations.

Figure 8.5: Experiential Learning Cycle (After Kolb 1984)

Both of these cycles have relevance for the types of models of training discussed in this chapter. In an AIDS counselling course, it may be useful to help trainees to reflect on their concrete experience of working in the AIDS field, to share those reflections in plenary sessions and then to develop models of counselling and methods of application. An addition, in the AIDS counselling workshop, would be formal theoretical inputs. As we have noted, one of the things that marks out AIDS counselling is the need to have up-to-date information about the disease. This formal input (via lectures or other didactic methods) can precede the use of the experiential learning cycle.

Malcolm Knowles, the American adult educator (1980) took a different approach to the definition of experiential learning. He described the activities that took place within the concept and thus listed the following, which he called 'participatory experiential techniques' :

- group discussion,
- cases,
- critical incidents,
- simulations,
- role-play,
- skills practice exercises,
- field projects,
- action projects,
- laboratory methods,
- consultative supervision (coaching),
- demonstrations,
- group seminars,
- work conferences,

- counselling,
- group therapy,
- community development (Knowles 1980)

Knowles' list seems so all-inclusive that he seems to have been saying that experiential learning techniques were any techniques other than the didactic lecture method or private, individual study and that experiential learning was synonymous with participant and discovery learning. To summarise the position adopted by those writers who devised their definitions of experiential learning from the work of Dewey, would involve noting first the accent on some sort of cycle of events starting with concrete experience. It is worth noting that Kolb's and Pfeiffer and Goodstein's cycles were, in fact, anticipated by Dewey himself:

> 'Thinking includes all of these steps, the sense of a problem, the observation of conditions, the formation and rational elaboration of a suggested conclusion and the active experimental testing.' (Dewey : 1916).

The notion of learning from experience being a cycle involving action and reflection was a theme frequently echoed amongst modern writers (see, for example : Kelly 1970, Hampden Turner 1966). Kolb's notion of transformation of experience and meaning can also be traced back to Dewey. He wrote that :

> 'In a certain sense every experience should do something to prepare a person for later experiences of a deeper and more expansive quality. That is the very meaning of growth, continuity, reconstruction of experience,' (Dewey 1938).

This, them, was the influence on experiential learning from the Dewey perspective. The accent, throughout, was on the primacy of personal experience and on reflection as the tool for changing knowledge and meaning. Again, given the personal nature of the AIDS field, it is important that workshop participants are encouraged to reflect on their own experiences, values and beliefs, throughout AIDS counselling training.

The particular characteristics of experiential learning

It is possible to draw out those characteristics that go to make up the approach to learning known as the experiential approach. These characteristics are offered as a further means of clarification and as the beginning of practical guidelines about how to use the approach in practice and in the context of organising and facilitating AIDS counselling workshops.

In experiential learning there is an accent on action

Both the Dewey and the humanistic approaches to experiential learning involve the learner in action. This is not to say that the learner is 'doing something' in a trivial sense but that she is engaged in an activity that should lead to learning. This is in opposition to traditional teaching/learning strategies which require that the learner remain passive in relation to an active teacher who is the dispenser of knowledge. Freire (1972) has called this traditional approach the 'banking' approach to education : knowledge is delivered to the learner in chunks and the learner later cashes out this information in examinations. The experiential learning approach is closer to Freire's concept of 'problem posing' education. Here, problems are encountered through discussion, argument and action. The learner is not longer passive but in dialogical relationship with an equally active teacher.

There is a second, less important sense of action too. In experiential learning the learner is often physically moving to take part in structured activities, role play, psychodrama and so on, as opposed to more traditional learning situations in which the learner is sat behind a desk or table. The application of this issue in the AIDS counselling workshop setting is clear : participants should be encouraged to 'try out' counselling skills in the safe setting of the workshop before they venture into the 'real world' of AIDS counselling. No amount of lectures, alone, can make a person an effective counsellor : like all skills, counselling skills have to be practised. Also, the emphasis on action permeates all aspects of AIDS counselling in that a prime objective in AIDS counselling is for the counsellor to have an effect on the behaviour of the client. In other words, the counsellor expects the client to act on what is discussed in the counsellor/client relationship.

Learners are encouraged to reflect on their experience

Most writers acknowledge that experience alone is not sufficient to ensure that learning takes place. Importance is placed on the integration of new experience with past experience through the process of reflection (Kolb 1984, Kilty 1983, Freire 1972, Burnard 1990). Reflection may be an introspective act in which the learner alone integrates new experience with old. It may also be a group process whereby sense is made of an experience through group discussion. If reflection as a group activity is to be successful, the group leader is required to act as a group facilitator and may require special skills and knowledge. It is suggested that the skills associated with group facilitation are different to the skills associated with the usual processes of teaching in that the group facilitator takes a non-directive or non-authoritarian stance in relation to the learners. In a reflective group, the leader as facilitator is not ascribing meanings to experience nor offering explanations but allowing learners to do these things for themselves. The reflective group can be used in the AIDS counselling workshop to allow participants to consider their own views and values : particularly in the fields of sexuality and ethics.

A phenomenological approach is adopted by the facilitator

Phenomenology may be defined as the description of objects or situations without their being ascribed values, meanings or interpretations. Phenomenology as a philosophy was developed by Husserl (1931) and underpins the philosophical writings of the existentialists (Sartre 1956, Macquarrie 1973).

The facilitator who uses a phenomenological approach restricts himself to the use of description as a means of summarising what a learner has said and enables that learner to invest their her own learning with meaning. The 'valuing' process is left to the learner. It is the learner who ascribes meaning to what is going on in the learning environment and the facilitator's meanings are not automatically foisted on the student. Reflecting this phenomenological approach, which eschews interpretation of experience by another person, Carl Rogers (1983) prefers to use the term 'facilitator of learning' rather than the more traditional terms 'teacher' or 'leader'. In using such a descriptor he hoped to remove the connotation of the teacher as expert or authority in the interpretation of experience. In the literature on experiential learning, the term facilitator is often used in preference to the terms teacher, lecturer, tutor or leader. In the context of AIDS counselling, this facilitative aspect of the trainers role is a crucial one in encouraging would-be counsellors to examine their own feelings and experiences in the fields of sexuality, beliefs and values.

There is an accent on subjective human experience

Alfred North Whitehead (1933) discussed the problem of 'dead knowledge' and asserted that knowledge kept no better than fish! The experiential approach to learning stresses the evolving, dynamic nature of knowledge. Rather than evoking R.S. Peter's (1972) notion of education as initiation in to particular ways of knowing, it stresses the importance of the learner understanding and creating a view of the world in that learner's own terms. Postman and Weingartner (1969) noted that traditional education assumes a linear model of knowledge in which there is absolute truth and a single fixed reality. Citing anthropological evidence that our language tends to limit our view of reality (Worf 1956) and that the means buy which subject matter is communicated fundamentally alters the content of that communication.

Experiential learning allows for different means of communicating concepts, accounts for 'multiple realities' and invites critical reflection. In this respect, it differs considerably from the traditional model of education and training.

Human experience is valued as a source of learning

The accent in experiential learning, through its variety of learning methods and through it's name, is on experience. Learners, as has been noted, are encouraged to reflect on past experiences to plan for future events. In formulating his concept of andragogy (the theory and practice of the education of adults), Malcolm Knowles (1978, 1980) stresses the value of experience in the sphere of adult learning. He maintains that as an individual matures so she accumulates an expanding reservoir of experience that causes her to become a rich resource for learning. Knowles argues that the resource should be tapped in the educational process because, as Knowles puts it : 'To an adult, his experience is who he is (Knowles 1978). Thus, for Knowles, there is an important ontological issue : an adult's experience is not something exterior and tacked on but is part of the person's self-concept. Experiential learning then is an attempt to make use of human experience as part of the learning process. It may be noted that the humanistic approach to experiential learning pays particular attention to the emotional aspect of the individual's experience (Heron 1981). The human element is clearly central in AIDS counselling. No workshop on AIDS counselling can afford to omit reference to the personal experience of the people present.

Finally, whilst discussing the characteristics of experiential learning it may be noted that what is under consideration is :

a) a set of teaching/learning methods and
b) an attitude towards learning.

It is important, too, to locate the experiential learning approach in an historical and cultural context. Given its roots in humanistic and student-centred learning methods, it may be so located as having its genesis in the 1960's and in the USA (Rogers 1983). It is also notable, that it has much in common with the client-centred approach to counselling, discussed throughout this book, in that it encourages the teacher or trainer to take the lead in the learning encounter from the student rather than to assume the more traditional role of the teacher as the person who hands on knowledge.

Thus experiential learning applied to the teaching of AIDS counselling can be both a set of teaching and learning methods to convey the knowledge and skills involved in learning how to become an AIDS counsellor and an attitude towards teaching those knowledge and skills that honours and respects personal experience and personal beliefs and values. It should be noted, though, that implicit in the experiential approach is also a set of values concerned with subjective experience, the valuing of individual learning and the centrality of the individual in the learning encounter. Whether or not such an individualistic approach is always appropriate in teaching and learning about AIDS remains an important point for discussion.

Limitations of this study

This study has identified some perceptions of AIDS counsellors and other professionals working in the field or in the related health care field. Given that it is a descriptive study, generalisation is impossible. It is not suggested that the findings in this study can be generalised out to a larger population of counsellors or health care professionals. On the other hand, interviews were continued until no new themes appeared to emerge. In this sense it can be tentatively suggested that some of the issues discussed by the respondents in this study would probably be discussed by other people too.

One particular limitation of the study was the nature of the sample. It was a mixed sample of both AIDS counsellors and health professionals. In that respect, it was not a 'clean' sample of one particular sort of person. This, however, was intentional : the aim was to get a broad range of perceptions from different sorts of people. Another study, however, might study only the perceptions of AIDS counsellors. Yet another might explore the perceptions of those people who receive AIDS counselling.

A criticism may be raised about asking people to identify how other people view the person with AIDS. In this study, respondent's were often asked how they imagined the person in the street may view the person with AIDS. Again, this was intentional : the aim was to explore how AIDS counsellors and health professionals felt their clients were viewed by others. Another researcher might ask the person in the street for his or her views directly.

A constant anxiety, throughout the study, was whether or not the researcher had read widely enough or had identified key papers in the field. Whilst this is every researcher's problem to some degree, it is highlighted in a project concerned with AIDS for material dates quickly and new papers are published with such frequency that no researcher could expect to keep up.

It would have been useful to extend the study to explore a wider range of people's perceptions, perhaps through the generation of a questionnaire for surveying a larger sample. It is the researcher's intention to continue the research in this way.

No study can claim to be in any way definitive. Another researcher, looking through different eyes, in a different cultural context would probably draw different conclusions from the data. It is a myth to believe that the 'data can speak for themselves'. All data analysis in the qualitative field involves judgements about what to include and what to leave out, how to categorise and what conclusions to draw after the analysis. It is hoped, however, that the current study offers some different perspectives on the issues of AIDS counselling and AIDS counselling training.

Implications for further research

Given the limitations described above and reviewing the findings of the study described here, it is possible to identify areas for further research. Some of these might be :

- The person with AIDS' perception of AIDS counselling,
- The person in the streets' perception of AIDS,
- The appropriateness of applying the principles of client-centred counselling to the AIDS field,
- The long term effect of giving out information about AIDS in terms of behaviour change,
- The effectiveness of AIDS counselling,
- The preferred styles of counselling used by AIDS counsellors.
- The AIDS counselling relationship : its implications for both counsellors and clients,
- The counselling needs of the person who is bisexual. This is a group that seems little addressed in the AIDS counselling literature and also in the research literature (Wolff 1977, Klein and Wolf 1986).
- The support systems that are or could be used by AIDS counsellors,
- The effectiveness of Six Category Intervention Analysis as a strategy for AIDS counselling.

Summary

This book has offered a review of some of the literature on AIDS counselling. It has described and reported a descriptive study of 21 respondents who were interviewed and whose responses were analysed using two different methods. It has concluded that there may be clear differences between 'ordinary' counselling and AIDS counselling but that AIDS counselling is a relatively young activity which may grow and develop as the AIDS field changes. The book has closed with some suggestions for training drawn from the research findings and from the literature on interpersonal skills training, counselling training and the adult learning and experiential learning literature.

Appendix I
Data analysis and the freeform database

In this appendix, the freeform database program is described as a tool which can help in at least two aspects of the research cycle : as part of the maintenance of a referencing system and as a tool for analysing qualitative data. Both aspects of the freeform database where used in the research project described in this book.

Fixed form databases

The more familiar database program for IBM compatible PC's is the fixed form database. There are numerous examples of these, ranging from *dbase*, to *Paradox* to *PC-File*. Some are expensive, large and quite difficult to learn. Others (such as *PC-File*) are fairly simple to use, very extensive in their range of operations and available as shareware. Shareware is a system of marketing that appears to be unique to computer software.

With shareware, the user pays a small fee to a company to cover the cost of the disk, the copying of the program and the postage and in return gets a fully functioning copy of the program. He or she can then try out the program before deciding whether or not to continue using it. If he or she does decide to keep the program, then he or she is asked to pay a registration fee to the writer of the program. This registration fee is nearly always much less than can be paid for standard, commercial packages (Hughes 1991).

The fixed form database requires that the user first makes some decisions about the type of data that is to be stored. For example, the person who chooses to store bibliographic references in such a database must first decide how may 'fields' he or she will require. A field is part of the screen that will contain specific information. In this example, separate fields will be used to store the following sorts of information : author; year; title and publisher.

Having decided on the sorts of fields that are required, the user must then decide how large each field will be. That is to say, that a decision must be made about the number of characters that will be typed into each of the fields. In the example here, there will be little trouble in deciding that only four characters will be needed for the 'year' field. Problems may arise in other fields. For example, how long is the longest title of a book or a journal article likely to be? It is often difficult, prior to using such a database, to decide on how little or how much space to allocate to each field.

The program usually has limits on the numbers of characters that can be placed in any given field. Usually this is quite a limitation : many programs only allow 250 characters to be entered into any field as a maximum. If the user wants to type in 'notes' or an 'abstract' at the bottom of each bibliographic reference, only 250 characters will be available for this purpose. Note, too, that 'characters' refers to single letters or spaces and should not be confused with 'words'. Figure 1 illustrates an example entry screen from a fixed form database. The broken lines within each 'field' represent the number of characters that can be entered. Normally, the field labels ('field 1' etc.) would not be shown : the are used here to illustrate the notion of a field.

Field 1 : **Author**	Field 2 **Year** :
Field 3 : **Title** :	
Field 4 : **Publisher (or Journal)**	
Field 5 : **Location** :	
Field 6 : **Keywords** :	
Field 7 : **Comments**:	

Figure 1 : Example of a Screen From a Fixed Form Database

Despite these limitations, the fixed form database has many advantages. It offers a systematic way of filing away information that can easily be retrieved from the computer. Searches can be run on a number of words or phrases. For example, it can be quite possible to search a bibliographic database of many thousands of entries for all of the journal articles written on counselling in psychiatric nursing, by British authors, between 1981 and 1983.

The fixed form database also allows the operator to browse through the data in much the same way as someone might browse through a drawer full of reference cards. Overall, the use of a computerised, fixed form database can do much to increase the efficiency of anyone who needs to keep a bibliographic database. That must include all nurse educators and most students.

The free form database

The fixed form database, as we have seen, imposes certain restrictions on the user. The free form database has few of these. Essentially, the free form database allows the operator to enter data in any format from the keyboard and makes no restriction on the number or types of fields. In other words, one database entry may contain three lines of type : another may contain two pages. In fact there is no concept of 'fields' with the free form database. The operator merely types in data and decides when one entry is complete. Figure 2 illustrates a typical screen from a free form database entry, this time with the text already in place.

It will be noted from figure 2 that because the free form database does not depend on fields nor upon fields of particular length, the user is free to write references into it in the standard 'Harvard' referencing style (Turk and Kirkman 1989).

> Heron, J. 1990 *Helping the Client* : Sage, London.
>
> This is an updated and more general version of the author's previous work : Six Category Intervention Analysis (published by the Human Potential Research Project, University of Surrey, Guildford). The six categories are :
>
> - Prescriptive,
> - Informative,
> - Confronting,
> - Cathartic,
> - Catalytic,
> - Supportive.
>
> There are copies of this in the library and it is useful to refer to both this and earlier editions.
>
> KEYWORDS : Interpersonal Skills, Counselling, Therapy.
>
> See various research projects which have used the Six Category approach as a format for identifying nurses' interpersonal skills.
>
> My copy lent to John Smith 18/1/91 : Check return!

Figure 2 : Example of a Free Form Database Screen

With the free form database, it is possible to recall any entry merely by recalling one word or phrase of the text in that entry. Imagine, for example, that the operator has typed in a large entry about a book on midwifery training. She recalls that the entry makes reference to 'didactic teaching'. To recall the entry to the screen, she uses the program to find the phrase 'didactic teaching' and this will be sufficient to recall the entry.

Alternatively, she remembers the author of the book : that, too, will be sufficient to find the reference. If all else fails, she can browse through all the entries until she finds the correct one.

The free form database is useful as a method of storing items of data of varying lengths and of different sorts. Anything from addresses, to bibliographic references to quotes from essays can be filed away in this sort of database and readily found again. Examples of this type of database are *Memory Mate*, *Agenda*, *Info Select* and *Ask Sam* (which may be best know as the program which was used to take down and structure the information relating to the American Irangate trial). As with fixed form databases, they range in price from around £30 to as much as £500 per program.

The free form database in research

Two applications of the free form database can be described. The applications described here have both been used by the author in the current research project. The database used in this case was Memory Mate (Fremont 1988), which is available for about £59 and also as shareware (when it is usually called *Instant Recall.*) The shareware version is rather less complete and versatile than the full cost program.

The program is very easy to use, very comprehensive in its documentation. Apart from its applications in the ways described here, it is also useful for the building of hypertext documents, for storing addresses and telephone numbers, for use as an 'ideas file' and so forth.

A hypertext feature also allows the user to read short sections of text and then to switch to other pages for more details of a particular concept (Beard 1991). Consider, for example, the following passage:

> Counselling in nursing has been developed in a variety of ways. Some writers describe the role of the nurse-as-counsellor, whilst

other writers discuss counselling skills. Both verbal and non-verbal skills are involved in counselling.

In a hypertext document, the computer user could stop on any of the italicised words in the above passage, press a button and be taken straight to more details about the topic in question. The hypertext approach allows for greater freedom and variety in the learning process. The free form database system allows for the development of such a system which has a considerable range of possible applications in the field of nurse education.

References

Perhaps the most immediate application of this sort of database program is as a means of storing bibliographic references. Because of the free form format of the program, no restrictions occur regarding the method or style of entry of the references. Thus, it is quite possible to store away summaries, quotes and notes alongside the details of the author, year, title and publisher.

It is also a simple matter to add to a particular entry at a later date. It becomes possible to develop a very useful and detailed database of references and notes. Further, with the use of the hypertext function, it becomes possible to link together all of the references on a particular topic or to link together various sorts of topics.

An important feature of *Memory Mate* is that it is a 'terminate and stay resident' program. That is to say that it can be called to the screen 'over' another program, worked on and then removed from the screen. Such programs are sometimes known as 'pop-up' programs because of their ability to pop up over the 'regular' program that is in use. This increases the program's usefulness. It becomes possible, for example, whilst working on an essay or paper (using a wordprocessing program) to check a reference whilst writing the paper (from the pop up database).

It is also possible to 'cut and paste' references from the pop-up database into the main program. Thus, when a reference list is being compiled at the end of the paper, all of the references can be pulled straight out of the database and place at the end of the paper. Thus less typing is involved and fewer mistakes are likely to occur. Plus, of course, a considerable amount of time is saved.

Finally, the cut and paste feature can be used in reverse. As a reference is used in an essay, it can be pasted directly into the database for further use at a later date. Paragraphs of information from documents used in the wordprocessor can also be transferred in this way.

For the researcher, the free form approach to bibliographic storage has other uses. First, it is useful to anyone who is carrying out a meta-analysis of the literature in a particular domain. The meta-analysis is a method of identifying a detailed range of literature and then subjecting it to a form of content analysis, in order to identifying the sorts of papers that have been written on a particular topic. Thus it becomes possible, when doing a meta-analysis of the counselling literature in nursing, to identify the numbers of papers in particular years, the ones that were written about psychiatric nursing, the ones that describe counselling skills and so on.

The free form database is particularly useful here. The researcher merely identifies the categories of the analysis (skills, year, theories etc,) and then runs searches through the database using those categories as keywords. The program will not only identify each occurrence of each keyword but will also identify the number of occurrences. Very quickly, a list of frequencies of occurrences of certain items can be drawn up.

As we noted above, the free form database has no notion of fields through which to search for items. Any item that is requested will be searched for through the whole of each data entry in the database. This ensures that any search that is run is exhaustive of the whole content of the database. This cannot so readily be achieved with a fixed form database.

Data analysis

The second application for the researcher is the use of the free form database as a tool for content analysis of interview data (Carney 1982, Berg, 1989). Here, the interviews are transcribed and entered into the database as single 'items'. It any item is too large, it can be divided up into manageable chunks, according to the limitations of the program. The transcripts can be readily prepared in any wordprocessor and transferred to the database in the form of ASCII files.

Once the transcripts are in the database, the researcher identifies his or her categories of search. For example, the person researching attitudes towards dying and who has used the interview method, may want to search through the data for examples of reference to Kubler - Ross's work (Kubler - Ross 1969). In this case, the name 'Kubler - Ross' is used as a keyword and the program searches through all of the data and identified both all of the occurrences of those two words and also the number of times that the words were used. Also, and most importantly, the program allows the researcher to see the use of the name Kubler - Ross in context. The program allows the enquirer to see each example of the use of the name, within the interview transcript itself. It should be noted, though, that the words Kubler - Ross must contain the hyphen if they are to be found. As ever, computers are only logical and concrete - they cannot anticipate mistakes or 'guess' at what is required. The development of 'fuzzy logic' or the ability for computers to guess in this way is being undertaken at the present time but not yet widely available. The GIGO ('garbage in : garbage out') principle still applies (Gosling 1982).

The searches for keywords in interview transcripts are not restricted to one or two words. Strings of words can be searched for. For example, the researcher may want to find out how often and in what context, the expression 'unconditional positive regard' (Rogers 1967) was used by respondents. Strings of words of this sort pose no problem. The only restriction, of course, is that the program will only find exact matches for the phrase. Thus, 'non-conditional regard' would be missed.

Whilst 'fuzzy logic' is not yet available in such programs, it is possible to execute 'wildcard' searches. This means that if the enquirer is not quite sure of the whole of a particular word, the program will still search for varieties of part of the word. For example, the command '**conditional' will call up examples of both 'unconditional' and 'inconditional', thus allowing for mistakes to be allowed for.

The free form database can quickly allow access to a wide range of approaches to content analysis. Words, phrases, dates, frequencies, repetitions and many more 'items' can be quickly and easily accessed. The fact that all of the items remain in context and are viewed as part of the original transcript make validity checks more possible (Burnard and Morrison 1990; Field and Morse 1985).

An alternative and even tighter method of analysis involves breaking down each paragraph in interview transcripts and importing each of these into the database as separate items. This is easily done and further ensures that each example of a particular word or phrase is counted effectively.

Overall, the free form database seems to have some specific advantages over the fixed form version, for the nurse educator, student and researcher. Easy data entry in any format, quick searching of all of the items in the database and frequency counts of searched-for items makes this type of program an almost essential one for anyone who uses a IBM compatible computer. Data processing for any researcher is an issue that needs careful thought - especially when datasets are large (Innes 1984). Whilst content analysis and similar forms of analysis can be carried out by hand, it seems reasonable to use the appropriate technology when it is available.

Apart from these programs, there is also purpose built software for analysing research data in nursing, ranging from SPSS/PC, a program which allows detailed statistical analysis of numerical data (which can, of course, be derived from coded interview data), to The Ethnograph : a large scale 'cut and paste' program which allows for the collation of items within pre-specified categories. Whilst the later is useful in grounded theory type projects (Glaser and Strauss 1967), the former is clearly not so useful in analysing qualitative data. Also, both of these programs need to be learned before they can be used. One of the advantages of the free form database program is that it is both easy to use and to become accustomed to.

It is quite possible to use both fixed form and the free form database programs. I find it useful to maintain a fixed form database as a cumulative bibliographic reference database. I add references to it in the same way that a person may write out a new reference card. This now contains nearly 1000 references of different sorts. It is frequently re-indexed in order to put it in alphabetical order, by author and items can be searched for on any one or more of the following keywords : author, title, publisher or keyword.

For current research and writing work, I use the free form data base which holds references and notes relating to a number of projects. This means that I can have almost instant access to a range of information ranging from fragments of ideas, to excerpts from papers, to contemporary references. I also find it useful for jotting down notes in much the same way as one might use 'Post-it' stickers, as reminders of various sorts.

Memory Mate is available direct from Express Technology Inc. 7655 East Gelding Drive, Scottsdale, Arizona 85260 USA. Phone, direct from UK : 1-800-98-1073.

Appendix II
Counsellor attitude scale

Name...............................Date.....................
Course...

After considering each statement, indicate whether or not you are in basic agreeement (A), disagreement (D) or cannot decide (?) by encircling the appropriate letter in the left-hand margin. Do not use (?) unless absolutely necessary. While there is no time limit, do not spend too much time pondering any one item.

A D ? 1. The counsellor's goal is to make people better adjusted to society.

A D ? 2. It is not the job of the counsellor to solve the client's problems.

A D ? 3. A thorough diagnosis is unnecessary for effective counselling.

A D ? 4. After the first interview the counsellor should plan each interview before meeting the client.

A D ? 5. In the counselling hour the client may discuss any area of concern he wishes.

A D ? 6. The counsellor should be in control of the interview at all times.

A D ? 7. The best way to understand the client is to compare him with other people.

A D ? 8. Whether the client requests it or not, the counsellor should suggest reading material pertinent to his problems.

A D ? 9. In order for the client to benefit most from the counselling experience he must be given unconditional acceptance by the counsellor.

A D ? 10. If the client is unable to understand his problem, the counsellor should explain it to him carefully and clearly.

A D ? 11. The function of the counsellor is to create and maintain an atmosphere in which the client may explore his feelings and attitudes in any way he wishes.

A D ? 12. The client must first establish a dependency relationship upon the counsellor before he can become independent.

A D ? 13. The counsellor does not have the right socially or professionally to allow a client to choose an inadequate or antisocial solution to his problem.

A D ? 14. The counsellor should always be the one to determine when counselling should be terminated.

A D ? 15. Each client has within himself the capacities to work out a solution to his problems without manipulation by the counsellor.

A D ? 16. If the counsellor has some negative feelings toward the counsellee in the initial interview, he should firmly but gently refuse to continue with him.

A D ? 17. If counselling is to be successful, the counsellor must depend, for the most part, on the client's own potential for growth.

A D ? 18. A complete case history is unnecessary before the counsellor actually begins counselling with the client.

A D ? 19. The counsellor should permit the client to solve his problems in his own way.

A D ? 20. The client has the right to consider and possibly choose goals that are antisocial or immoral.

A D ? 21. In the counselling interview the client has the right to say anything he wishes about the counsellor.

A D ? 22. The counsellor should offer the client advice when it is clearly needed.

A D ? 23. The best way of understanding the client is to try to see him as he sees himself.

A D ? 24. In the final analysis people must work out their own solutions to their problems.

A D ? 25. If the counsellor talks about a number of problems at the same time the counsellor should tell him to concentrate on one problem at a time.

A D ? 26. The counsellor should praise the client whenever appropriate.

A D ? 27. One of the counsellor's main functions is to try to convey to the client that he accepts the client's feelings and attitudes.

A D ? 28. After the client has decided upon his goals the counsellor should tell him how he can achieve them.

A D ? 29. When a client feels his situation is hopeless the counsellor should not try to reassure him.

A D ? 30. When the client does not understand the meaning of a particular piece of behaviour the counsellor should explain it to him.

A D ? 31. The counsellor should not permit the client to express attitudes which are contrary to his own in the field of ethics, religion, politics etc.

A D ? 32. When the counsellor feels that the client is making a mistake he should not try to discourage him.

A D ? 33. The counsellor should ask questions only when he does not understand what the client has said.

A D ? 34. If the client presents a point of view that is obviously prejudiced or distorted, the counsellor should set him straight.

A D ? 35. Verbalisation of insight is not crucial in counselling.

A D ? 36. After a therapeutic working relationship has been established the counsellor should begin to interpret the client's unconscious attitudes and feelings.

A D ? 37. If a client announces his intentions of performing a criminal act, the counsellor should discourage him.

A D ? 38. The counsellor's main function is to provide a thoroughly accepting and permissive atmosphere in which the client may work out his problems if he desires.

A D ? 39. After a client has stated his problem the counsellor should offer one or more possible solutions to serve as a basis for further discussion.

A D ? 40. Early in the counselling process the counsellor should reassure the client that his problem is not insoluble and thereby reduce his anxiety so he can start working on his problems.

A D ? 41. The counsellor should feel free to ask the client questions in order to obtain pertinent information necessary for the solution of the client's problem.

A D ? 42. If a client wants to discontinue counselling he should be allowed to do so.

A D ? 43. When the counsellor sees that the client is solving his problems realistically he should praise and encourage the client.

A D ? 44. If the client's life situation demands an immediate decision, or some course of action, and the client feels unable to make a choice, the counsellor should make suggestions.

A D ? 45. If the client wishes to spend long periods in silence, the counsellor should let him.

A D ? 46. If a client threatens suicide, the counsellor should endeavour to help the client explore his underlying feelings.

A D ? 47. The counsellor should end each interview with some word of reassurance.

A D ? 48. The counsellor should give advice when the client requests it.

A D ? 49. A formal verbal structuring of the counselling relationship should occur in the first interview.

A D ? 50. Client resistance should not be interpreted to the client but merely accepted.

A D ? 51. In the initial contact with the client the counsellor should develop a friendly social relationship as a basis for counselling.

A D ? 52. The counsellor should not assume the major responsibility for the content of discussion during the counselling.

A D ? 53. Most clients are unable to take the responsibility for the solution to their problems; otherwise they would not be in counselling.

A D ? 54. The major contribution of the counsellor to the solution of the client's problem is the providing of an objective, external point of view.

A D ? 55. The client should be allowed to indulge in self-pity.

A D ? 56. The counsellor should discourage long pauses in counselling to keep the client from feeling embarrassed of uncomfortable.

A D ? 57. When a client seems to be unable to talk about himself, the counsellor should engage in 'small talk' to get him started.

A D ? 58. It is rarely helpful for the counsellor to let the client know what he would when faced with the same problem.

A D ? 59. The purpose of the first interview with a client is to get a survey of the nature of the client's problem.

A D ? 60. If the counsellor feels the client persists in wasting interview time, he should share his feelings with the client.

A D ? 61. The counsellor should try to help the client see his problem in a logical way.

A D ? 62. The counsellor should never take a client's statements at face value, since the client is not aware of the hidden import behind them.

A D ? 63. The counsellor should be objective and impersonal in his relationship with the client.

A D ? 64. The more information the counsellor has about the client prior to the counselling interview, the better he will be able to understand the client.

A D ? 65. When the client veers away from the discussion of a significant problem area, he should always be brought back to it in a gentle, subtle or round-about way by the counsellor.

A D ? 66. The successful counsellor is one who is able to suggest solutions to the client's problems in such a way that the client feels they are his own.

A D ? 67. The counsellor should allow the client to make self-derogatory statements.

A D ? 68. When the client makes conflicting statements, the counsellor should try to get at the true facts in the situation.

A D ? 69. It is unnecessary for the counsellor to obtain a clear picture of the nature and origins of the client's problem before he can help him/her.

A D ? 70. The counsellor should refrain from adapting the counselling relationship to the expectations of the client.

Counselling Skills Attitude Scale : Scoring Key.

1. D
2. A
3. A
4. D
5. A
6. D
7. D
8. D
9. A
10. D
11. A
12. D
13. D
14. D
15. A
16. D
17. A
18. A
19. A
20. A
21. A
22. D
23. A
24. A
25. D
26. D
27. A
28. D
29. A
30. D
31. D
32. A
33. A
34. D
35. A
36. D
37. D
38. A
39. D
40. D
41. D
42. A
43. D
44. D
45. A
46. A
47. D
48. D
49. D
50. A
51. D
52. A
53. D
54. D
55. A
56. D
57. D
58. A
59. D
60. A
61. D
62. D
63. D
64. D
65. D
66. D
67. A
68. D
69. A
70. A

The Counsellor Attitude Scale was developed in 1972 by Dr Richard Nelson-Jones and Professor C.H. Patterson and used and reproduced with permission.

References

A.A.H.P. 1962 Articles of Association : Association for Humanistic Psychology : San Francisco, California.

Acevedo, J.R. 1989 A Group Model for AIDS Prevention and Support. In Dilley, J.W., Pies, C. and Helquist, M. : Face to Face : A Guide to AIDS Counselling : AIDS Health Project, University of California, San Francisco, California.

Adler, A. 1927 The Practice and Theory of Individual Psychology : Harcourt, Brace, Jovanovitch, New York.

Aggleton, P. 1989 Evaluating health education about AIDS. In P. Aggleton, G. Hart and P. Davies (eds) : AIDS : Social Representations, Social Practices : Falmer Press, Lewes.

Alberti, R.E. and Emmons, M.L. 1982 Your Perfect Right : a Guide to Assertive Living : Impact, San Luis Obispo, California.

Andersen, H. and MacElveen-Hoen, P. 1988 Gay clients with AIDS : new challenges for hospice programs : Hospice Journal : Physical, Psychosocial and Pastoral Care of the Dying : 4 : 2 : 37 - 54.

Anderson, H.H. (ed) 1959 Creativity and Its Cultivation : Harper and Row, New York.

Aronson, E. 1980 The Social Animal : 3rd Edition : Freeman, San Francisco, California.

Bailey, C.R. 1983 Experiential Learning and the Curriculum : Nursing Times : July 20th : 45 - 46.

Ball, M.J., Hannah, K.J., Gerdin Jelger, U. and Peterson, H. (eds) 1988 Nursing Informatics : Where Nursing and Technology Meet : Springer Verlag, New York.

Bandura, A. 1990 Perceived Self-Efficacy in the Exercise of Control over AIDS Infection : Evaluation and Program Planning : 13 : 9 - 17.

Barnes, D.M. 1983 Teaching Communication Skills to Student Nurses - an Experience : Nurse Education Today : 13 : 2 : 45 - 48.

Barrick, B. 1989 Teaching safer sex : a nursing intervention in the AIDS epidemic : Imprint : 36 : 1 : 51 - 53.

Beard, N. 1991 Computing Common Sense : Personal Computer World : 14 : 3 : 243 - 244.

Berg, B.L. 1989 Qualitative Research Methods for the Social Sciences : Allyn and Bacon, New York.

Blake, R. and Mouton, J. 1976 The D/D Matrix : Scientific Methods. Cited in Heron, J. 1986 Six Category Intervention Analysis : Human Potential Research Project, University of Surrey, Guildford.

Bond, S., Rhodes, T.J. 1990 HIV infection and community midwives : knowledge and attitudes Midwifery : 6 : 1 : 86 - 92.

Bond, M. 1986 Stress and Self-Awareness : A Guide for Nurses : Heinemann, London.

Bor, R. 1991 The ABC of AIDS Counselling Nursing Times : 87 : 1 : 32 - 35.

Bor, R., Miller, R. and Salt, H. 1989 Secrecy Related Problems in AIDS Management : Journal of the Royal College of Physicians : 23 : 264 - 267.

Bor, R., Miller, R., Perry, L et al 1989 Strategies for counselling the 'worried well' in relation to AIDS : Journal of the Royal Society of Medicine : 23 : 218 - 220.

Boud, D.J. (ed) 1981 Developing Student Autonomy in Learning : Kogan Page, London.

Boudieu, P. 1971 Systems of Education and Systems of Thought. In M.F.D. Young : Knowledge and Control : New Directions for the Sociology of Education : Collier Macmillan, London.

Boydel T. 1976 Experiential Learning : Manchester Monograph No 5: Department of Adult and Higher Education, Manchester University.

Brown, Y., Calder, B., and Rae, D. 1990 The effect of knowledge on nursing students' attitudes toward individuals with AIDS : Journal of Nursing Education : 29 : 8 : 367 - 372.

Burgess, R.G. (ed) 1982 Field Research : A Sourcebook and Field Manual : Allen and Unwin, London.

Burgess, R.G. 1982 Elements of Sampling in Field Research. In R.G. Burgess (ed) Field Research : A Sourcebook and Field Manual : Allen and Unwin, London.

Burnard, P. 1990 Learning Human Skills : An Experiential Guide for Nurses : 2nd Edition : Heinemann, Oxford.

Burnard 1991 Experiential Learning in Action : Avebury, Aldershot.

Burnard, P. 1990 Learning Human Skills : 2nd Edition : Heinemann, Oxford.

Burnard, P. and Morrison, P. 1989 Counselling Attitudes in Community Psychiatric Nurses : Community Psychiatric Nursing Journal : 9 : 5 : 26 - 29.

Burnard, P. 1989 Teaching Interpersonal Skills : An Experiential Handbook for Health Care Professionals : Chapman and Hall, London.

Burnard, P. 1991 Experiential Learning in Action : Avebury, Aldershot.

Burnard, P. and Morrison, P. 1990 Nursing Research in Action : Developing Basic Skills : Macmillan, London.

Burnard, P. and Morrison, P. 1990 Counselling Attitudes in Health Visiting Students : Health Visitor : 63 : 11 : 389 - 390.

Burnard, P. and Morrison, P. 1990 Nursing Research in Action : Developing Basic Skills : Macmillan, London.

Burnard, P. and Morrison, P. 1988 Nurses' Perceptions of Their Interpersonal Skills : a Descriptive Study Using Six Category Intervention Analysis : Nurse Education Today : 8 :266 - 272.

Burnard, P. and Morrison, P. 1991 Client-Centred Counselling : A Study of Nurses' Attitudes : Nurse Education Today : 11 : 104 - 109.

Burnard, P. 1989 Counselling Skills for Health Professionals : Chapman and Hall, London.

Burnard, P. 1987 Spiritual Distress and the Nursing Response : Theoretical Considerations and Counselling Skills : Journal of Advanced Nursing : 12 : 377 - 382.

Burnard, P. and Morrison, P. 1988 Nurses' Perceptions of Their Interpersonal Skills : a Descriptive Study Using Six Category Intervention Analysis : Nurse Education Today : 8 :266 - 272.

Burnard, P. and Morrison, P. 1989 Counselling Attitudes in Community Psychiatric Nurses : Community Psychiatric Nursing Journal : 9 : 5 : 26 - 29.

Burnard, P. 1988 The Heart of the Counselling Relationship : Senior Nurse : 1988 : 8 : 12 : 17 - 18.

Carkuff, R. 1983 The Art of Helping : 5th Edition : Human Resources Development Press, Amherst, Mass.

Carney, J. 1982 Content Analysis : Harper and Row, London.

Clare, A. 1981 Let's Talk About Me : BBC, London.

Clare, A. with Thompson, S. 1981 Let's Talk About Me! : BBC, London.

Coccellari, A., Dilley, J.W. and Shore, M. 1988 Neuropsychiatric aspects of AIDS dementia complex : a report on a clinical series : Neurotoxicology : 9 : 381 - 390.

Connor, S. and Kingman, S. 1989 The Search for the Virus : The Scientific Discovery of AIDS and the Quest for a Cure : Penguin, Harmondsworth.

Cook, A., Fischer, G., Jones, E. et al 1988 Preventing AIDS Among Substance Abusers ; A Training for Substance Abuse Treatment Counsellors : The Center for AIDS and Substance Abuse Training : Falls Church, VA.

Cormier, L., Cormier, W. and Weisser, R. 1984 Interviewing and Helping Skills for Health Professionals : Wadsworth, Monterey, California.

D'Augelli 1989 AIDS fears and homophobia among rural nursing personnel : AIDS : Education and Prevention : 1 : 4 : 277 - 284.

Davis, H. and Fallowfield, L. (eds) 1991 Counselling and Communication in Health Care : Wiley, Chichester.

de Bono, E. 1970 Lateral Thinking : Penguin, Harmondsworth.

Dennis, H. 1991 Getting the Message : Nursing Standard : 5 : 17 : 55 - 56.

Denzin, N.K. 1970 The Research Act : Aldine, Chicago.

Dewey, J. 1916 Democracy and Education : Free Press,London.

Dewey, J. 1938 Experience and Education : Collier Macmillan, London.

Dietrich, G.C. 1978 Teaching of Psychiatric Nursing in the Classroom : Journal of Advanced Nursing : 3 : 525 - 534.

Dilley, J.W., Pies, C. and Helquist, M. Face to Face : A Guide to AIDS Counselling : AIDS Health Project, University of California, San Francisco.

Dilley, J.W., Pies, C. and Helquist, M. 1989 Face to Face : a Guide to AIDS Counselling : AIDS Health Project, University of California, San Francisco, California.

Dillman, D.A. 1978 Mail and Telephone Surveys : Wiley, New York.

DiMarzo, D. 1989 Double Jeopardy : Haemophilia and HIV Disease. In Donoghue, M., Stimson, G. and Dolan, K. 1989 Sexual behaviour of injecting drug users and associated risks of HIV infection for non-injecting sexual partners : AIDS Care : 1 : 51 - 58.

Dorn, F.J. 1984 Counselling as Applied Social Psychology : An Introduction to the Social Influence Model : Thomas, Springfield, Illinois.

Dorn, N. and South, N. 1990 Communication, Education, Drugs and HIV. In J. Strang and G. Stimson : AIDS and Drug Misuse : The Challenge for Policy and Practice in the 1990's : Routledge, London.

Driscoll, R. 1984 Pragmatic Psychotherapy : Van Nostrand Reinhold, New York.

Eakes, G.G. and Lewis, J.B. 1991 Should nurses be required to administer care to patients with AIDS? Students respond : Nurse-Educator 16 : 2: 36-8.

Egan, G. 1990 The Skilled Helper : A Systematic Approach to Effective Helping : 4th Edition : Books/Cole, Pacific Grove, California.

Egan, G. 1982 The Skilled Helper : 2nd Edition : Brooks/Cole, Monterey, California.

Ellis, A. and Dryden, W. 1987 The Practice of Rational-Emotive Therapy : Springer, New York.

Ellis, R. and Whittington, D. 1981 A Guide to Social Skills Training : Croom Helm, London.

Ellis, A. 1987 The Evolution of Rational-Emotive Therapy (RET) and Cognitive-Behaviour Therapy (CAB). In Zeig, J.K. (ed) : The Evolution of Psychotherapy : Brunner/Mazel, New York.

F.E.U. 1983 Curriculum Opportunity : A Map of Experiential Learning in Entry Requirements to Higher and further Education Award Bearing Courses : Further Education Unit, London.

Faltz, B.G. 1989 Strategies for Working With Substance Abusing Clients. In Dilley, J.W., Pies, C. and Helquist, M. Face to Face : A Guide to AIDS Counselling : AIDS Health Project, University of California, San Francisco.

Farrelly, F. and Brandsma, J. 1974 Provocative Therapy : Meta Publications, Cupertino, California.

Federal Centre for AIDS : 1987 Caring Together : The Report of the Expert Working Group on Integrated Palliative Care for Persons With AIDS : Federal Centre for AIDS, Health and Welfare, Canada.

Field, P.A. and Morse, J.M. 1985 Nursing Research : The Application of Qualitative Approaches : Croom Helm, London.

Fink, A and Kosekoff, J. 1985 How to Conduct Surveys : A step-by-step guide : Sage, Beverly Hills, California.

Fitzpatrick, M. and Milligan, D. 1990 Reflections on the AIDS panic : Living Marxism : 15 : 14 - 19.

Flaskerud, J.H. 1989 Psychiatric nurses' needs for AIDS information : Perspectives in Psychiatric Care : 25 : 3/4 : 3 - 9.

Folstein, M. 1984 AIDS anxiety in the 'worried well'. In Nichols, S.E., Ostrow, D.G. : Psychiatric Implication of Acquired Immune Deficiency Sydrome : American Psychiatric Press, Washington.

Frankenberg, R. 1990 Review article : Disease, literature and the body in the era of AIDS - a preliminary exploration : Sociology of Health and Illness : 12 : 3 : 351 - 359.

Freemont, M. 1989 Memory Mate : Broderbund Software, San Rafael, California.

Freire, P. 1972 Pedagogy of the Oppressed : Penguin, Harmondsworth.

Fromm 1979 To Have or to Be? : Abacus Books, London.

Fromm, E. 1957 The Art of Loving : Unwin, London.

Fullilove, M.T. 1989 Ethnic Minorities, HIV disease and the growing underclass. In J.W. Dilley, C. Pies and M. Heliquist : Face to Face : A Guide to AIDS Counselling : AIDS Health Project, University of California, San Francisco, California.

Gauch, R.R., Feeney, K.B. and Brown, J.W. 1990 Fear of AIDS and attrition among medical technologists: American Journal of Public Health : 80 :10: 1264-5

Gaze, H. 1987 Keep morals out : religious attitudes to AIDS : Nursing Times : 83 : 50 : 16 - 29.

George, H. 1989 Counselling People With AIDS, Their Lovers, Friends and Relations. In Green, J. and McCreaner, A. (eds) Counselling in HIV Infection and AIDS : Blackwell, London.

Getzels, J.W. and Jackson, P.W. 1962 Creativity and Intelligence : Wiley, Chichester.

Giglioli, P. (ed) 1982 Language and Social Context : Penguin, Harmondsworth.

Gilchrist, L.D. and Schinke, S.P. 1983 Coping With Contraception : Cognitive and Behavioural Methods With Adolescents : Cognitive Therapy and Research : 7 : 5 : 379 - 388.

Glaser, B.G. and Strauss, A.L. 1967 The Discovery of Grounded Theory : Aldine, New York.

Goble, J. 1990 Psychodrama Takes Centre Stage : Nursing Times : 86 : 28 : 34 - 35.

Goldblum, P.B. and Moulton, J. 1989 HIV Disease and Suicide. In Dilley, J.W., Pies, C. and Helquist, M. : Face to Face : A Guide to AIDS Counselling : AIDS Health Project, University of California, San Francisco, California.

Goldenberg, D. and Laschinger, H. 1991 Attitudes and normative beliefs of nursing students as predictors of intended care behaviors with AIDS patients: a test of the Ajzen-Fishbein Theory of Reasoned Action : Journal of Nursing Education : 30 : 3 : 119 - 126.

Gonen, J.Y. 1971 The Use of Psychodrama Combined with Videotaped Playback on an In-Patient Floor : Psychiatry : 34 : 198 - 213.

Gosling, P.E. 1982 Mastering Computer Programming : Macmillan, London.

Green, J. 1989b Post - Test Counselling. In Green, J. and McCreaner, A. (eds) Counselling in HIV Infection and AIDS : Blackwell, London.

Green, J. 1989 Counselling in Developing Countries. In Green, J. and McCreaner, A. (eds) Counselling in HIV Infection and AIDS : Blackwell, London.

Green, J. and Sherr, L. 1989 Dying, Bereavement and Loss. In Green, J. and McCreaner, A. (eds) Counselling in HIV Infection and AIDS : Blackwell, London.

Groat, L. 1982 Meaning in Post-Modern Architecture : An Examination Using the Multiple Sorting Task : Journal of Environmental Psychology : 2 : 3 : 3 - 22.

Grossman, R. 1985 Some Reflections on Abraham Maslow : Journal of Humanistic Psychology : 25 : 4 : 31 -34.

Hall, C. 1984 A Primer of Freudian Psychology : Mentor Books, New York.

Hampden-Turner, C. 1966 An Existential Learning Theory : Journal of Applied Behavioural Science : 12 : 4 : 36 - 43.

Hancock, C. 1991 AIDS Focus : The Challenge for Nurses : Nursing Standard : 5 : 17 : 50 - 52.

Heath, J. 1983 Gaming/Simulation in Nurse Education : Nurse Education Today : 13 : 4 : 92 - 95.

Heidegger, M. 1927 Being and Time : Harper and Row, New York.

Heron, J. 1977 Behaviour Analysis in Education and Training : Human Potential Research Project : University of Surrey, Guildford.

Heron, J. 1989 Helping the Client : Sage, London.

Heron, J. 1986 Six Category Intervention Analysis : Human Potential Research Project, University of Surrey, Guildford.

Heron, J. 1978 Co-Counselling Teachers Manual : Human Potential Research Project, University of Surrey, Guildford.

Heron, J. 1986 Six Category Intervention Analysis : 2nd Edition : Human Potential Research Project : University of Surrey, Guildford.

Heron, J. 1977 Catharsis in Human Development : Human Potential Research Project : University of Surrey, Guildford.

Heron, J. 1981 Paradigm Papers : Human Potential Research Project : University of Surrey, Guildford.

Heron, J. 1973 Experiential Training Techniques : Human Potential Research Project, University of Surrey, Guildford.

Hopper, L., Jesson, A. and Macleod Clark, J. 1991 Progression to Counselling : Nursing Times : 87 : 8 : 41 - 43.

Horney, K. 1937 The Neurotic Personality of Our Time : Norton, New York.

Howard, G.S., Nance, D.W. and Myers, P. 1987 Adaptive Counselling and Therapy : A Systematic Approach to Selecting Effective Treatments : Jossey-Bass, San Francisco.

Howe, J. 1989 AIDS - The rights approach : Professional Nurse : 5 : 3 : 156 - 159.

Hughes, K. 1991 What is Shareware? : PC Shareware Magazine : 1 : 3 : 7.

Hugman, R. 1991 Power in Caring Professions : Macmillan, London.

Hurtig, W. and Fandrick, C. 1990 The nursing student and the psychiatric patient with AIDS : a case study : Nurse Education Today : 10 : 2 : 92 - 97.

Husserl, E. 1931 Ideas : General Introduction to Pure Phenomenology : trans G. Boyce : Allen and Unwin, London.

Innes, A.E. 1984 Data Processing for Business Studies : 2nd Edition : Macdonald and Evans, Plymouth.

Ivey, A.E. 1991 Developmental Strategies for Helpers : Individual, Family and Network Interventions : Brooks/Cole, Pacific Grove, California.

Jackins, J. 1970 The Fundamentals of Co-Counselling Manual :Rational Island Publishers, Seattle, Washington.

Jackins, H. 1965 The Human Side of Human Beings : Rational Island Publishers, Seattle, Washington.

James, W. 1902 The Varieties of Religious Experience : Random House, Toronto.

Jarvis, P. 1984 The Theory and Practice of Adult and Continuing Education : Croom Helm, London.

Johnson, A. and Gill, O. 1989 Evidence for recent changes in the sexual behaviour of homosexual men. Phil. Trans. R. Soc. Lond. : B325 : 153 - 61.

Jung, C.G. 1931 Modern Man In Search of a Soul : Rascher, Zurich.

Kagan, C., Evans, J. and Kay, B. 1986 A Manual of Interpersonal Skills for Nurses : An Experiential Approach : Harper and Row, London.

Keeton, M. and Associates 1976 Experiential Learning : Jossey Bass, San Francisco, California.

Kelly, G. 1955 The Psychology of Personal Constructs : Volumes 1 and 2 : Norton, New York.

Kilty, J. 1983 Experiential Learning : Human Potential Research Project, University of Surrey, Guildford.

Kim, M.J., McFarland, G.K. and McLance, A.M. 1987 Pocket Guide to Nursing Diagnoses : 2nd edition : C.V. Mosby, St Louis, Missouri.

Kirby, D. 1985 The Effects of Shcool Education Programs : A Review of the Literature : Journal of School Health : 50 : 559 - 563.

Kirkman, C. and Turk, J. 1989 Effective Writing : Improving Scientific, Technical and Business Communication : Spon, London.

Kirkpatrick, W. 1988 AIDS : Sharing the Pain : Pastoral Guidelines : Darton, Longman and Todd, London.

Kirschenbaum, H. 1979 On Becoming Carl Rogers : Dell, New York.

Kitzinger, J. 1990 Audience understandings of AIDS media messages : a discussion of methods : Sociology of Health And Illness : 12 : 3 : 319 - 335.

Klein, F. and Wolf, T. 1986 Two Lives to Lead : Bisexualities : Theory and Practice : Harrington Park Press, London.

Klonoff, E,A and Ewers,D. 1990 Care of AIDS patients as a source of stress to nursing staff : AIDS-Education-and-Prevention : 2 : 4 : 338-48.

Knowles, M.S. 1978 The Adult Learner : A Neglected Species : 2nd Edition : Gulf, Texas.

Knowles, M.S. 1980 The Modern Practice of Adult Education : From Pedagogy to Andragogy :2nd Edition : Follett, Chicago.

Knox, M.D., Dow,M.G., and Cotton, D.A. 1989 Mental health care providers: the need for AIDS education : AIDS Education and Prevention : 1 :4 : 285-90.

Koch, R. and Rankin, J. (eds) 1987 Computers and Their Application in Nursing : Harper and Row, London.

Kok, G.J. 1990 The Effectiveness of Sexual Education for Young People. In P.C. Liedekerken, R. Jonkers, W.F.M. de Haes, G.J. Kok and H. Saan (eds) Effectiveness of Health Education : Van Gorcum, Assen, Netherlands.

Kolb, D. 1984 Experiential Learning : Prentice Hall, Englewood Cliffs, New York.

Kubler-Ross, E. 1969 On Death and Dying : Tavistock, London.

Last, J.M. 1988 Natural and Social History of Epidemics : AIDS : A Perspective for Canadians : Background Papers : Royal Society of Canada, Ontario.

Leukefeld, C.G. 1988 AIDS counselling and testing : Health and Social Work : 13 : 3 : 167 - 169.

Lewis, C.E. and Montgomery, K. 1990 : The AIDS-related experiences and practices of primary care physicians in Los Angeles: 1984-89 : American Journal of Public Health 80 : 12 : 1511-3.

Logan, J.C. 1971 Use of Psychodrama and Sociodrama in Reducing Negro Aggression : Group Psychotherapy and Psychodrama : 24 : 138 - 149.

Lovejoy, N.C. and Moran, T.A. 1988 Selected AIDS beliefs, behaviours and informational needs of homosexual/bisexual men with AIDS or ARC : International Journal of Nursing Studies : 25 : 3 : 207 - 216.

MacCaffrey, E.A. 1987 Counselling AIDS patients : a unique approach by Shanti therapists : AIDS Patient Care : 1 : 2 : 26 - 27.

Macks, J. 1989 The Psychological Needs of People with AIDS. In Dilley, J.W., Pies, C. and Helquist, M. : Face to Face : A Guide to AIDS Counselling : AIDS Health Project, University of California, San Francisco, California.

Macquarrie, J. 1973 Existentialism : Penguin, Harmondsworth.

Mahrer, A.L. 1989 A Case of Fundamentally Different Existential-Humanistic Psychologies : Journal of Humanistic Psychology : 29 : 2 : 249 - 261.

Marshall, T.A. and Nieckarz, J.P. 1988 Bereavement Counselling : AIDS Patient Care : 2 : 2 : 21 - 25.

Marson, S.N. 1979 Nursing : a Helping Relationship? : Nursing Times : March 29th : 541 - 544.

Maslach, C. 1981 Burnout : The Cost of Caring : Prentice Hall, New Jersey.

Maslow, A. 1972 Motivation and Personality : 2nd Edition : Harper and Row, London.

Masson, J. 1990 Against Therapy : Fontana, London.

May, R. 1989 Answer to Ken Wilber and John Rowan : Journal of Humanistic Psychology : 29 : 2 : 244 - 248.

McCreaner, A. 1989c Training Models. In Green, J. and McCreaner, A. (eds) Counselling in HIV Infection and AIDS : Blackwell, London.

McCreaner, A. 1989 Pre-Test Counselling. In Green, J. and McCreaner, A. (eds) Counselling in HIV Infection and AIDS : Blackwell, London.

McGough, K.N. 1990 Assessing social support for people with AIDS : Oncology Nursing Forum : 17 : 1 : 31 - 35.

McNulty, M. 1984 A Framework for the Future : Nursing Mirror : 158 :9 : pages not numbered.

Miller, D. 1987 Living With AIDS and HIV : Macmillan, London.

Miller, C. 1990 The AIDS Handbook : Penguin, Harmondsworth.

Miller, D. 1986 How to Counsel Patients About HIV Disease - Those Who Have It and Those Who Fear It : Maternal and Child Health : 11 : 10 : 322 - 30.

Miller, R., Goldman, E., Bor, R. et al 1989 Counselling Children and Adults About AIDS/HIV : Counselling Psychology Quarterly : 2 : 65 - 72.

Miller, R. and Bor, R. 1990 Counselling for HIV Screening in Women. In Studd, J. (ed) Progress in Obstetrics and Gynaecology : Churchill Livingstone, Edinburgh.

Moreno, J.L. 1969 Psychodrama : Volume three : Beacon House Press, Beacon, New York.

Moreno, J.L. 1977 Psychodrama : Volume one : 4th Edition : Beacon House Press, Beacon, New York.

Moreno, J.L. 1959 Psychodrama : Volume two : Beacon House Press, Beacon, New York.

Morrison, P. and Burnard, P. 1991 Caring and Communicating : The Interpersonal Relationship in Nursing : Macmillan, London.

Murgatroyd, S. 1985 Counselling and Helping : Methuen, London.

Murphy, G. and Kovach, J.K. 1972 Historical Introduction to Modern Psychology : 6th Edition : Routledge and Kegan Paul, London.

Murphy, J., John, M. and Brown, J. 1984 Dialogues and Debates in Social Psychology : Open University Press, Milton Keynes.

Nelkin, D. 1987 AIDS and the social sciences : review of useful knowledge and research needs : Review of Infectious Diseases : 9:947 - 60.

Nelson-Jones, R. 1981 The Theory and Practice of Counselling Psychology : Holt, Rhinehart and Winston, London.

Nelson-Jones, R. 1981 The Theory and Practice of Counselling Psychology : Holt, Rhinehart and Winston, London.

Off Pink Collective 1988 Bisexual Lives : Off Pink Collective, London.

Palmer, R. and Pope, C. 1984 Brain Train : Studying for Success : Spon, London.

Perls, F. 1973 The Gestalt Approach and Eyewitness to Therapy : Science and Behaviour Books, Palo Alto, California.

Perry, S. and Tross, S. 1984 Psychiatric problems of AIDS inpatients at the New York Hospital : a Preliminary Report : Public Health Reports : 99 : 200 - 205.

Peters, R.S. 1972 Education as Initiation. In R.D. Archambault(ed) Philosophical Analysis and Education : Routledge and Kegan Paul, London.

Pfeiffer, J.W. and Goodstein, L.D. 1982 The 1982 Annual for Facilitators, Trainers and Consultants : University Associates, San Diego, California.

Pines, A.M., Aronson, E. and Kafry, D. 1981 Burnout : From Tedium to Personal Growth : Free Press, New York.

Postman, N. and Weingartner, C.W. 1969 Teaching as a Subversive Activity :Penguin, Harmondsworth.

Pratt, R.J. 1988 AIDS : A Strategy for Nursing Care : Arnold, London.

Pye, M., Kapila, M., Buckley, G. and Cunningham, D. (eds). 1989 Local AIDS Programmes in the UK : Longman, London.

Quilliam, S. and Grove-Stephensen, I. 1981 The Best Counselling Guide : Thorsons, London.

Reed, E.J. 1984 Using Psychodrama With Critical Care Nurses : Dimensions of Critical Care Nursing : 3 : 2 : 110 - 114.

Richardson, M., Bishop, J., Caygill, D., Mace, C., Ross, R, Taylor, S. and Tuczemskyi, E. 1990 : Disabled for a Day : Nursing Times : 86 : 21 : 66 - 67.

Richmond, V. McCroskey, J. and Payne, S. 1987 Nonverbal Behaviour in Interpersonal Relations : Prentice Hall, Englewood Cliffs, New Jersey.

Roffman, R.A. et al 1990 Continuing unsafe sex : assessing the need for AIDS prevention counselling : Public Health Reports : 105 : 2 : 202 - 208.

Rogers, C.R. 1983 Freedom to Learn for the Eighties : Merrill, Columbus, Ohio.

Rogers, C.R. 1951 Client-Centred Therapy : Constable, London.

Rogers, C.R. 1952 Client Centred Therapy : Constable, London.

Rogers, C.R. 1972 The Facilitation of Significant Learning. In M.L. Silberman, J.S. Allender and J.M. Yanoff : The Psychology of Open Teaching and Learning : Little Brown, Boston.

Rogers, C.R. 1967 On Becoming a Person : Constable, London.

Rogers, C.R. 1983 Freedom to Learn for the Eighties : Merrill, Columbus, Ohio.

Rogers, C.R. 1970 On Encounter Groups : Penguin, Harmondsworth.

Rogers, C.R. 1986 Reflection of Feelings : Person-Centred Review : 2 : 375 - 377.

Rowan, J. 1989 The Self : One or Many? The Psychologist : Bulletin of the British Psychological Society : : 7 : 279 - 281.

Rowan, J. and Dryden, W. 1989 Innovative Therapy in Britain : Open University Press, Milton Keynes.

Rowntree, G. (ed) 1987 Fundamentals of Computing : NCC Publications, Manchester.

Sartre, J-P, 1955 Being and Nothingness : Philosophical Library : New York.

Schallma, H, Kok, G., Braeken, D., Shopman, M. and Deven, F. 1991 Sex and AIDS Education for Adolescents : Tijdschrift voor Seksuologie : 15 : 140 - 149.

Schulman, D. 1982 Intervention in Human Services : A guide to skills and knowledge : 3rd Edition : C.V. Mosby : St Louis, Missouri.

Siegel, J. and Scipio-Skinner, K.V. 1983 Psychodrama : an Experiential Model for Nursing Students : Group Psychotherapy, Psychodrama and Sociometry : 36 : 97 - 101.

Silven, D. and Caldarola, T.J. 1989 The HIV-Positive Client. In J.W. Dilley, C. Pies and M. Helquist : Face to Face : A Guide to AIDS Counselling : AIDS Health Project, University of California, San Francisco, California.

Silverman, D. and Perakyla, A. 1990 AIDS counselling : the interactional organisation of talk about 'delicate' issues : Sociology of Health and Illness : 12 : 3 : 293 - 317.

Simon, S, Howe,E. and Kirschenbaum, H. 1978 Values Clarification : 2nd Edition : A & W Visual Library, New York.

Sketchley, J. 1989 Counselling people affected by HIV and AIDS. In W. Dryden, D.Charles-Edwards and R. Woolfe : Handbook of Counselling in Britain : Tavistock/Routledge, London.

Spradley, J.P. 1979 The Ethnographic Interview : Holt, Rinehart and Winston, New York.

Stedeford, A. 1989 Counselling, Death and Bereavement. In Dryden, W., Charles-Edwards, D. and Woolfe, R. (eds) Handbook of Counselling in Britain : Routledge, London.

Stevens, J.O. 1971 Awareness : Exploring, Experimenting, Exploring : Real People Press, Moab, Utah.

Strang, J. and Stimpson, G. (eds) 1990 AIDS and Drug Misuse : The Challenge for Policy and Practice in the 1990's : Routledge, London.

Sue, S. and Zane, N. 1987 The role and cultural techniques in psychotherapy : a critique and reformulation : American Psychologist : 42 : 37 - 45.

Swanson, J.M., Chenitz,C., Zalar, M. and Stoll, P. 1990 A critical review of human immunodeficiency virus infection- and acquired immunodeficiency syndrome-related research: the knowledge, attitudes, and practice of nurses : Journal of Professional Nursing 6 : 6: 341-55.

Tschudin, V. 1991 Counselling Skills for Nurses : 3rd Edition : Balliere Tindall, London.

Van Ments, M. 1983 The Effective Use of Role-Play : Kogan Page, London.

Vroome, E.M.M., Paalman, M.E.M, Sandfort, Th.G.M., Sleutjes, M., deVrieds, K. and Tileman, R.A.P. 1990 AIDS in the Netherlands : the effects of several years of campaigning : International Journal of STD and AIDS : 1 : 268 - 275.

Walker, R. (ed) 1985 Applied Qualitative Research : Gower, Aldershot.

Warner-Robbins, C.G. and Christiana, N.M. 1989 The spiritual needs of persons with AIDS : Family and Community Health : 12 : 2 : 43 - 51.

Watkins, R. and Addison, J. 1990 All the World's a Stage : Nursing Times : 86 : 21 : 47 - 48.

Weinstein, M., Crayton, E. and Goodjoin, R. 1989 Black Sexuality : A Bibliography : 2nd Edition : MIRA Publications, San Francisco.

Welch, J. and Newbury, J. 1990 Looking After People with Late HIV Disease : The Patten Press in association with the Lisa Sainsbury Foundation.

Wellings, K. and Wadsworth, J. 1990 AIDS and the moral Climate. In Jowell, R, Witherspoon, S. and Brooks, L. (eds) British Social Attitudes : the 7th Report : Gower, Aldershot.

Whitehead, A.N. 1933 The Aims of Education : Benn, London.

Wibley, S. 1983 The Use of Role Play : Nursing Mirror : June 22nd : 54 - 55.

Wills, D.J. 1990 A survey of nurses attitudes to AIDS related issues : New Zealand Nursing Forum : 18 : 4 : 7 - 9.

Wolff, C. 1977 Bisexuality : a Study : Quartet, London.

Worf, B.J. 1956 Language, Thought and Reality : Selected Writings : Technology Press of Massachusetts Institute of Technology : Cambridge, Mass.

Yalom, I.D. 1977 Existential Psychotherapy. In O.L. McCabe (ed) Changing Human Behaviour : Grune and Stratton, New York.

Yelin, E.H., Greenblatt, R.M., Hollander, H. and McMaster J.R. : 1991 : The impact of HIV-related illness on employment : American Journal of Public Health : 81 : 1 : 79-84.

Youngman, M.B. 1978 Designing and Analysing Questionnaires : Nottingham University School of Education, Nottingham.

Bibliography

Adams-Webber, J. and Mancusco, J.C. (eds) Applications of Personal Construct Theory : Academic Press, London.

Adler, R.B., Rosenfield, L.B. and Towne, N. 1983 Interplay : The Process of Interpersonal Communication : Holt, Rinehart and Winston, London.

Adler, R.B. and Towne, N. 1984 Looking Out/Looking In : Interpersonal Communication : Holt Rinehart and Winston, London.

Adler, R. and Rodman, G. 1988 Understanding Human Communication : 3rd Edition : Holt, Rinehart and Winston, New York.

Adler, R.B. 1977 Confidence in Communication : A Guide to Assertive Social Skills : Holt Rinehart and Winston, London.

Aggleton, P. 1989 Evaluating health education about AIDS. In P. Aggleton, G. Hart and P. Davies (eds) : AIDS : Social Representations, Social Practices : Falmer Press, Lewes.

Alberti, R. (ed) 1977 Assertiveness : Innovations, Applications, Issues : Impact, San Luis, Obispo, California.

Alberti, R.E. and Emmons, M.L. 1982 Your Perfect Right : A Guide to Assertive Living : 4th Edition :Impact Publishers, San Luis, California.

Alderman, C. 1991 AIDS : Changing Times Nursing Times : 5 : 17 : 53 - 54 .

Altman, D. 1986 AIDS and the New Puritanism : Pluto Press, London.

Andersen, H. and MacElveen-Hoen, P. 1988 Gay clients with AIDS : new challenges for hospice programs : Hospice Journal : Physical, Psychosocial and Pastoral Care of the Dying : 4 : 2 : 37 - 54.

Argyle, M. 1983 The Psychology of Interpersonal Behaviour : 4th Edition : Penguin, Harmondsworth.

Argyle, M (ed) 1981 Social Skills and Health : Methuen, London.

Argyris, C. and Schon, D. 1974 Theory in Practice : Increasing Professional Effectiveness : Jossey Bass, San Francisco.

Argyris, C. 1982 Reasoning, Learning and Action :Jossey Bass, San Francisco.

Armitage, P. and Burnard, P. 1991 Mentors or Preceptors? Narrowing the Theory-Practice Gap : Nurse Education Today : 11 : 225 - 229.

Arnold, E. and Boggs, K. 1989 Interpersonal Relationships : Professional Communication Skills for Nurses :Saunders, Philadelphia.

Ashworth, P. and Morrison, P. (1991) Problems of competence-based nurse education. Nurse Education Today, 11, 256-260.

Ausberger, D. 1979 Anger and Assertiveness in Pastoral Care : Fortress Press, Philadeplphia.

Baer, J. 1976 How to Be Assertive (Not Aggressive) : Women in Life, in Love and on the Job : Signet, New York.

Bailey, R. and Clarke, M1989 Stress and Coping in Nursing

Chapman and Hall.

Bailey, R. 1985 Coping With Stress in Caring :Blackwell, Oxford.

Baker, R. 1984 Stress in Welfare Work : National Children's Home, Occasional Papers. No 5 : 1 - 24.

Bannister, D. and Fransella, F. 1986 Inquiring Man : 3rd Edition : Croom Helm, London.

Barrick, B. 1989 Teaching safer sex : a nursing intervention in the AIDS epidemic : Imprint : 36 : 1 : 51 - 53.

Baruth, L.G. 1987 An Introduction to the Counselling Profession :Prentice Hall, Englewood Cliffs, New Jersey.

Belkin, G.S.1984 Introduction to Counselling :Brown, Dubuque, Iowa.

Bellack, A.S. and Hersen, M (eds) : 1979 Research and Practice in Social Skills Training : Plenum Press, New York.

Benner, P. and Wrubel, J. 1989 The Primacy of Caring : Stress and Coping in Health and Illness :Addison Wesley, Menlo Park.

Berg, B.L. 1989 Qualitative Research Methods for the Social Sciences : Allyn and Bacon, New York.

Berliner, H. 1984 AIDS and the Hospice : Health Service Journal : 98 : 424.

Bertrand, J.T., Makani, B., Hassig, S.E., Niwembo, K.L., Djunghu, B. and Muanda, M. 1991 AIDS Related Knowledge, Sexual Behaviour and Condom Use Among Men and Women in Kinshasa, Zaire : American Journal of Public Health : 81 : 3 : 53 - 58.

Bolger, A.W. (ed) 1982 Counselling in Britain : a reader: Batsford Academic, London.

Bond, S., Rhodes, T.J. 1990 HIV infection and community midwives : knowledge and attitudes Midwifery : 6 : 1 : 86 - 92.

Bond, J. 1991 Experience and Preparation of Community Nursing Staff for Work Associated With HIV Infection and AIDS : Social Science and Medicine : 32 : 1 : 71 - 76.

Bond, M. and Kilty, J. 1986 Practical Methods of Dealing With Stress : 2nd Edition :Human Potential Research Project,University of Surrey, Guildford.

Boone, E.J., Shearon, R.W., White, E.E. and Associates 1980 Serving Personal and Community Needs Through Adult Education :Jossey Bass, San Francisco, California.

Bor, R., Miller, R., Perry, L et al 1989 Strategies for counselling the 'worried well' in relation to AIDS : Journal of the Royal Society of Medicine : 23 : 218 - 220.

Boud, D., Keogh, R. and Walker, M. 1985 Reflection : Turning Experience into Learning :Kogan Page, London.

Boud, D. and Prosser, M.T. 1980 Sharing Responsibility : Staff-Student Cooperation in Learning :British Journal of Educational Technology : 11 : 1 : 24 -35.

Bower, S.A. and Bower, G.H. 1976 Asserting Yourself : Addison Wesley : Reading, Mass.

Bower, S.A. and Bower, G.H. 1976 : Asserting Yourself : Addison Wesley : Reading, Mass.

Boydel, E.M. and Fales, A.W. 1983 Reflective Learning : Key to Learning From Experience :Journal of Humanistic Psychology : 23 : 2: 99-117.

Bram, P.J. and Katz, L.F. 1989 A Study of Burnout in Nurses Working in Hospice and Hospital Oncology Settings : Oncology Nursing Forum : 16 : 4 : 555 - 560.

Brasweel, M. and Seay, T.1984 Approaches to Counselling and Psychotherapy Waverly, Prospect Heights.

Broome, A. 1990 Managing Change : Macmillan, London.

Brown, D. and Srebalus, D. J. 1988 An Introduction to the Counselling Process Prentice Hall, Philadelphia, PA.

Brown, S.D. and Lent, R.w. (eds) 1984 Handbook of Counselling Psychology Wiley, Chichester.

Bryman, A. 1988 Quantity and Quality in Social Research : Unwin Hyman, London.

Buber, M. 1958 I and Thou : Scribner, New York.

Bucknall, A. 1988 AIDS and Injecting Drug Users : The Practitioner : 232 : 463 - 466.

Bugental, E.K. and Bugental, J.F.T. 1984 Dispiritedness : a new perspective on a familiar state : Journal of Humanistic Psychology : 24 : 1 : 49 - 67.

Bugental, J.F.T. 1980 The far Side of Despair : Journal of Humanistic Psychology : 20 : 49 - 68.

Burgess, R.G. (ed) 1982 Field Research : A Sourcebook and Field Manual : Allen and Unwin, London.

Burnard, P. 1987 Nurse Education in the USA : Senior Nurse : 7 : 5 : 27 - 38.

Burnard, P. 1984 Training to Be Aware : Senior Nurse : 1 : 23 : 25 - 27.

Burnard, P. 1987 Nurse Educators and Experiential Learning : Nursing Times : 84 : 2 : 56.

Burnard, P. 1987 Teaching the Teachers : Nursing Times : 83 : 49 : 63 - 65.

Burnard, P. 1987 Developing Skills as a Group Facilitator : The Professional Nurse : 3 : 1 : 19 - 21.

Burnard, P. 1987 Interpersonal Skills : Sharing a Viewpoint : Senior Nurse : 7 : 3 : 38 - 39.

Burnard, P. and Morrison, P. 1987 Nurses' Perceptions of Their Interpersonal Skills : Nursing Times : 83 : 42 : 59.

Burnard, P. 1987 Counselling Skills : Journal of District Nursing : 6 : 7 : 12 - 14.

Burnard, P. 1984 Counselling the Counsellors : Senior Nurse : 1 : 13 : 15 - 19.

Burnard, P. 1987 The Health Visitor as Counsellor : a Framework for Interpersonal Skills : Health Visitor : 60 : 8 : 269.

Burnard, P. 1987 The Right Direction : Senior Nurse : 7 : 1 : 30 - 32.

Burnard, P. 1985 How to Reduce Stress : Nursing Mirror : 16 : 19 : 47 - 48.

Burnard, P. 1987 Learning to Listen : Journal of District Nursing : 6 : 9 : 26 - 28.

Burnard, P. 1988 Communicating on the Telephone : Senior Nurse : 8 : 13 : 14 - 18.

Burnard, P. 1988 Developing Counselling Skills in Health Visitors : an Experiential Approach : Health Visitor : 61 : 5 : 20 - 23.

Burnard, P. 1988 Self-Awareness : Journal of District Nursing : 6 : 10 : 27 - 29.

Burnard, P. 1988 Emotional Release : Journal of District Nursing : 6: 11 : 26 - 28.

Burnard, P. 1986 Encountering Adults : Senior Nurse : 4 : 4 : 30 - 31.

Burnard, P. 1989 Exploring Nurse Educators' Views of Experiential Learning : a Pilot Study : Nurse Education Today : 9 : 1 : 39 -45.

Burnard, P. 1987 Spiritual Distress and the Nursing Response : Theoretical Considerations and Counselling Skills : Journal of Advanced Nursing : 12 : 377 - 382.

Burnard, P. 1987 Meditation : Uses and Methods in Psychiatric Nurse Education : Nurse Education Today : 7 : 4 : 191 - 197.

Burnard, P. 1989 Developing Critical Ability in Nurse Education : Nurse Education Today : 9 : 271 - 275.

Burnard, P. 1991 The Language of Experiential Learning : Journal of Advanced Nursing : 16 : 7 : 873 - 879.

Burnard, P. 1984 The Human Potential Movement : a Personal Perspective : Self and Society : The European Journal of Humanistic Psychology : xii : 2 : 28 - 34.

Burnard, P. 1983 Through Experience and From Experience : Nursing Mirror : 156 : 9 : 29 - 33.

Burnard, P. 1987 Towards an Epistemological Basis for Experiential Learning : Journal of Advanced Nursing : 12 : 189 - 193.

Burnard, P. 1986 Psychiatric Nurse Education : a Question of Balance? : Nurse Education Today : 6 : 215 - 218.

Burnard, P. 1988 'Brainstorming' : A Practical Learning Activity in Nurse Education : Nurse Education Today : 8 : 354 - 358.

Burnard, P. 1988 Experiential Learning : Some Theoretical Considerations : International Journal of Lifelong Education : 7 : 2 : 127 - 133.

Burnard, P. 1988 Self-Awareness and Intensive Care Nursing : Intensive Care Nursing : 4 : 67 - 70.

Burnard, P. and Morrison, P. 1988 Nurses' Perceptions of Their Interpersonal Skills : a Descriptive Study Using Six Category Intervention Analysis : Nurse Education Today : 8 : 266 - 272.

Burnard, P. 1988 The Journal as an Assessment and Evaluation Tool in Nurse Education : Nurse Education Today : 8 : 105 - 107.

Burnard, P. 1986 Integrated Self-Awareness Training : a holistic model : Nurse Education Today : 6 : 219 - 222.

Burnard, P. 1987 Coping With Emotion in Intensive Care Nursing : Intensive Care Nursing : 3 : 4 : 157 - 159.

Burnard, P. 1988 Self Evaluation Methods in Nurse Education : Nurse Education Today : 8 : 229 - 233.

Burnard, P. 1984 The Way Forward : Senior Nurse : 1 : 12 : 14 - 18.

Burnard, P. 1989 Counselling Skills for Health Professionals : Chapman and Hall, London

Burnard, P. and Morrison, P. 1989 Counselling Attitudes in Community Psychiatric Nurses : Community Psychiatric Nursing Journal : 9 : 5 : 26 - 29.

Burnard, P. 1988 Coping With Other People's Emotions : The Professional Nurse : 4 : 1 : 11 - 14.

Burnard, P. 1989 Teaching Interpersonal Skills : An Experiential Handbook for Health Professionals : Chapman and Hall, London.

Burnard, P. 1988 The Spiritual Needs of Atheists and Agnostics : The Professional Nurse : 1988 : 4 : 3 : 130 - 132.

Burnard, P. 1989 Counselling in Surgical Nursing : Surgical Nurse : 2 : 5 : 12 - 14.

Burnard, P.1988 The Heart of the Counselling Relationship : Senior Nurse : 1988 : 8 : 12 : 17 - 18.

Burnard, P. 1990 Learning to Care for the Spirit : Nursing Standard : 4 : 18 : 38 - 39.

Burnard, P. 1989 Exploring Sexuality : Journal of District Nursing : 8 : 4 : 9 - 11.

Burnard, P. and Morrison, P. 1990 Nursing Research In Action L Developing Basic Skills : Macmillan, London.

Burnard, P.1988 The Spiritual Needs of Atheists and Agnostics : The Professional Nurse : 1988 : 4 : 3 : 130 - 132.

Burnard, P. 1987 Spiritual Distress and the Nursing Response :theoretical considerations and counselling skills :Journal of Advanced Nursing : 12 : 377 - 382.

Burnard, P. 1989 The Nurse as Non-Conformist : Nursing Standard : 4 : 1 : 32 - 35.

Burnard, P. 1990 Counselling the Boss : Nursing Times : 86 : 1 : 58 - 59.

Burnard, P. 1988 Preventing Burnout : Journal of District Nursing : 7 : 5 : 9 - 10.

Burnard, P. 1990 Learning Human Skills : An Experiential Guide for Nurses : 2nd Edition : Heinemann, Oxford.

Burnard, P. 1988 AIDS and Sexuality : Journal of District Nursing : 7 : 2 : 7 - 8.

Burnard, P. 1989 The 'Sixth Sense' : Nursing Times : 85 : 50 : 52 - 53.

Burnard, P. 1987 Counselling : Basic Principles in Nursing : The Professional Nurse : 2 : 9 : 278 - 280.

Burnard, P. 1987 Self and Peer Assessment : Senior Nurse: 6 : 5 : 16 - 17.

Burnard, P. 1987 Meaningful Dialogue : Nursing Times : 83 : 20 : 43 - 45.

Burnard, P. 1986 Hazard, Tutor at Work : Senior Nurse : 5 : 5 - 6.

Burnard, P. 1986 Picking Up the Pieces : Nursing Times : 82 : 17 : 37 - 39.

Burnard, P. 1985 Listening to People : Nursing Mirror : 16 :18 : 28 - 29.

Burnard, P. 1985 Teacher as Facilitator : Senior Nurse : 2 : 9 : 34 - 37.

Burnard, P. 1987 Playing the Game : Nursing Times : 13 : 61 - 62.

Burnard, P. 1988 Building on Experience : Senior Nurse : 8 : 5 : 18 - 20.

Burnard, P. 1989 Exploring Nurses' Attitudes to AIDS : The Professional Nurse : 5 : 2 : 84 - 90.

Burnard, P. 1988 The Heart of the Counselling Relationship : Senior Nurse : 1988 : 8 : 12 : 17 - 18.

Burnard, P. and Morrison, P. 1990 Counselling Attitudes in Health Visiting Students : Health Visitor : 63 : 11 : 389 - 390.

Burnard, P.1989 Existentialism as a Theoretical Basis for Counselling in Psychiatric Nursing Archives of Psychiatric Nursing : 3 : 3 : 142 - 147.

Burnard, P. 1987 Spiritual Distress and the Nursing Response :theoretical considerations and counselling skills : Journal of Advanced Nursing : 12 : 377 - 382.

Burnard, P. 1986 Learning About Groups : Nurse Education Today : 6 : 116 - 120.

Burnard, P. and Morrison, P. 1989 Counselling Attitudes in Community Psychiatric Nurses : Community Psychiatric Nursing Journal : 9 : 5 : 26 - 29.

Burnard, P. 1985 Learning to Communicate : Nursing Mirror : 16: 19 : 30 - 31.

Burnard, P. 1991 Teachers and Counsellors : Potential Role Conflict in the Workplace : Employee Counselling Today : 3 : 1 : 21 - 23.

Burnard, P. 1988 Searching for Meaning : Nursing Times : 84 : 37 : 34 - 36.

Burnard, P. 1988 No Need to Hide : Nursing Times : 84 : 24 : 36 - 38.

Burnard, P. 1988 Coping With Other People's Emotions : The Professional Nurse : 4 : 1 : 11- 14.

Burnard, P. 1988 AIDS and Sexuality : Journal of District Nursing : 7 : 2 : 7 - 8.

Burnard, P. 1988 Self-Directed Learning : Journal of District Nursing : 7 ;1; 7 - 8.

Burnard, P. 1988 Discussing Spiritual Issues With Clients : Health Visitor : 61 : 12 : 371 - 372.

Burnard, P. 1988 Empathy : The Key to Understanding : The Professional Nurse : 3 : 10 : 388 - 392.

Burnard, P. 1988 Preventing Burnout : Journal of District Nursing : 7 : 5 : 9 - 10.

Burnard, P. 1988 The Heart of the Counselling Relationship : Senior Nurse : 8 : 12 : 17 - 18.

Burnard, P. 1989 Psychiatric Nursing Students' Perceptions of Experiential Learning : Nursing Times : 85 : 1 : 52.

Burnard, P. 1991 Towards Enlightenment : Nursing Standard : 5 : 45 : 48 - 49.

Burnard, P. 1984 Developing Self-Awareness : Nursing Mirror : 158 : 21 : 30 -31.

Burnard, P. 1988 Mentors : a Supporting Act : Nursing Times : 84 : 46 : 27 - 28.

Burnard, P. 1988 The Spiritual Needs of Atheists and Agnostics : The Professional Nurse : 4 : 3 : 130 - 132.

Burnard, P. 1988 Equality and Meaning : Issues in the Interpersonal Relationship : Community Psychiatric Nursing Journal : 8 : 6 : 17 - 21.

Burnard, P. 1988 Stress and Relaxation in Health Visiting : Health Visitor : 61 : 12 : 272.

Burnard, P. 1989 Learning From the Learners : Nursing Standard : 4 : 6 : 26 - 27.

Burnard, P. 1989 The 'Sixth Sense' : Nursing Times : 85 : 50 : 52 - 53.

Burnard, P. 1989 Exploring Nurses' Attitudes to AIDS : The Professional Nurse : 5 : 2 : 84 - 90.

Burnard, P. 1989 The Nurse as Non-Conformist : Nursing Standard : 4 : 1 : 32 - 35.

Burnard, P. and Morrison, P. 1989 Client-Centred Approach : Nursing Times : 85 : 15 : 60 - 61.

Burnard, P. 1990 Counselling in Crises : Journal of District Nursing : 8 : 7 : 15 - 16.

Burnard, P. 1989 Exploring Nurses' Attitudes to AIDS : The Professional Nurse : 5 : 2 : 84 - 90.

Burnard, P. 1990 Recording Counselling in Nursing : Senior Nurse : 10 : 3 : 26 - 27.

Burnard, P. and Morrison, P. (1990) Psychological aspects of self-esteem. Surgical Nurse, 3, 4, 4-8.

Burnard, P. 1989 Exploring Sexuality : Journal of District Nursing : 8 : 4 : 9 - 11.

Burnard, P. 1989 Counselling in Surgical Nursing : Surgical Nurse : 2 : 5 : 12 - 14.

Burnard, P. 1990 Counselling in Crises : Journal of District Nursing : 8 : 7 : 15 - 16.

Burnard, P. 1990 Counselling the Boss : Nursing Times : 86 : 1 : 58 - 59.

Burnard, P. 1990 Staying in Balance : Humanistic Psychology and Psychiatric Nursing : Community Psychiatric Nursing Journal : 10 : 1 : 16 -19.

Burnard, P. 1989 The Role of Mentor : Journal of District Nursing : 8 : 3 : 8 - 10.

Burnard, P. and Morrison, P. 1989 Counselling Attitudes in Community Psychiatric Nurses : Community Psychiatric Nursing Journal : 9 : 5 : 26 - 29.

Burnard, P. 1990 Learning to Care for the Spirit : Nursing Standard : 4 : 18 : 38 - 39.

Burnard, P. 1991 Key Nursing Issues in AIDS Counselling : Nursing Times : 87 : 20 : 53.

Burnard, P. 1991 Students as Adults? : Nursing Standard : 5 : 35 : 44 - 46.

Burnard, P. and Morrison, P. 1990 Counselling Attitudes in Health Visiting Students : Health Visitor : 63 : 11 : 389 - 390.

Burnard, P. 1990 Using Experiential Teaching Methods : Nursing Times : 86 : 41 : 53.

Burnard, P. 1990 Recording Counselling in Nursing : Senior Nurse : 10 : 3 : 26 - 27.

Burnard, P. 1990 Stating the Case : Counselling : The Journal of the British Association for Counselling : 1 : 4 : 114 - 116.

Burnard, P. 1991 Exploring Personal Values : Journal of District Nursing : 9 : 7 : 7 - 8.

Burnard, P. 1990 Group Discussion : Nursing Times : 12 : 86 : 36 - 37.

Burnard, P. 1990 The Cult of the Personality : Nursing Standard : 5 : 14 : 46 - 47.

Burnard, P. 1985 Stop, Look and Listen. : Senior Nurse : 2 : 9 : 21 - 22.

Burnard, P. 1990 The Student Experience : Adult Learning and Mentorship Revisited : Nurse Education Today : 10 : 5 : 349 - 353.

Burnard, P. and Morrison, P. 1991 Client-Centred Counselling : A Study of Nurses' Attitudes : Nurse Education Today : 11 : 104 - 109.

Burnard, P. 1991 Using Video as a Reflective Tool in Interpersonal Skills Training : Nurse Education Today : 11 : 143 - 146.

Burnard, P. 1989 Experiential Learning and Andragogy - Negotiated Learning in Nurse Education : a Critical Appraisal : Nurse Education Today : 9 : 5 : 300 - 306.

Burnard, P. 1989 Existentialism as a Theoretical Basis for Counselling in Psychiatric Nursing : Archives of Psychiatric Nursing : III : 3 : 142 - 147.

Burnard, P. and Morrison, P. 1991 Nurses' Interpersonal Skills : a Study of Nurses' Perceptions : Nurse Education Today : 11 : 1 : 24 - 29.

Burnard, P. and Morrison, P. 1989 What is an Interpersonally Skilled Person? : A Repertory Grid Account of Professional Nurses' Views : Nurse Education Today : 9 : 6 : 384 - 391.

Burnard, P. 1991 Assertiveness and Clinical Practice : Nursing Standard : 5 : 33 : 37 - 39.

Burnard, P. and Morrison, P. 1990 Psychological Aspects of Self-Esteem : Surgical Nurse : 3 : 4 : 4 - 6.

Burnard, P. 1988 Four Dimensions in Counselling : Nursing Times : 84 : 20 : 37 - 39.

Burnard, P. 1991 Acquiring Minimal Counselling Skills : Nursing Standard : 5 : 46 : 37 - 39.

Burnard, P. 1990 Critical Awareness in Nurse Education : Nursing Standard : 4 : 30 : 32 - 34.

Burnard, P. 1988 Searching for Meaning : Nursing Times : 84 : 37 : 34 - 36.

Burnard, P. 1991 Perceptions of AIDS : Journal of District Nursing : 9 : 12 : 24 - 26.

Burnard, P. 1991 Improving Through Reflection : Journal of District Nursing : 9 : 11 : 10 - 12.

Burnard, P. 1991 Interpersonal Skills Training : Journal of District Nursing : 9 : 10 : 17 - 20.

Burnard, P. 1991 Changes in Theory, Language and Psychiatric Nursing : Nexus : The Journal of the Mental Health Network : 1 : 4 : 18 - 21.

Burnard, P. 1991 Beyond Burnout : Nursing Standard : 5 : 43 : 46 - 48.

Burnard, P. 1990 Ambivalence in Humanistic Psycholgy : Self and Society : The European Journal of Humanistic Psychology : XVIII : 3 : 40 - 41.

Burnard, P. 1990 Problems With M.E. : Journal of District Nursing : 8 : 12 : 22 - 23.

Burnard, P. 1991 Outpatient Object Lesson : Nursing Standard : 5 : 39 : 45 - 46.

Burnard, P. 1990 The Supervisory Role : Journal of District Nursing : July : 26 - 27.

Burnard, P. 1990 Is Anyone Here a Mentor? : Nursing Standard : 4 : 37 : 46.

Burnard, P. 1991 Perceptions of Experiential Learning : Nursing Times : 87 : 8 : 47.

Burnard, P. 1991 Peer Support Groups : Journal of District Nursing : 9 : 8 : 19 - 20.

Burnard,P. 1990 Exploring Meaninglessness : Journal of District Nursing : 9 : 6 : 10 - 13.

Calnan, J. 1983 Talking With Patients :Heinemann, London.

Campbell, A. 1984 Paid to Care? :S.P.C.K., London.

Campbell, A. 1984 Moderated Love :S.P.C.K., London.

Campbell, A.V. 1981 Rediscovering Pastoral Care :Darton, Longman and Todd, London.

Carkuff, R.R. 1969 Helping and Human Relations : Vol I :Selection and Training :Holt, Rinehart and Winston, New York.

Carr, P. 1991 HIV at Home : Home and Health Care Nursing : 9 : 2 : 45 - 46.

Carson B.V.1989 Spiritual Dimensions of Nursing Practice W.B. Saunders, Philadelphia.

Chenevert, M. 1978 Special Techniques in Assertiveness Training for Women in the Health Professions : C.V. Mosby, St Louis.

Chrousos, G.P., Loriaux, D.L. and Gold, P.W. 1988 Mechanisms of Physical and Emotional Stress : Plenum Press, New York.

Cianni-Surridge, M. and Horan, J. 1983 On the Wisdom of Assertive Job-Seeking Behaviour : Journal of Counselling Psychology : 30 : 209 - 214.

Clark, C. 1978 Assertive Skills for Nurses :Contemporary Publishing, Wakefield, Mass.

Clark, D. 1988 AIDS and the Family : 27th May : 21 - 22.

Coccellari, A., Dilley, J.W. and Shore, M. 1988 Neuropsychiatric aspects of AIDS dementia complex : a report on a clinical series : Neurotoxicology : 9 : 381 - 390.

Connor, S. and Kingman, S. 1989 The Search for the Virus : The Scientific Discovery of AIDS and the Quest for a Cure : Penguin, Harmondsworth.

Connor, S. and Kingman, S. 1989 The Search for the Virus : The Scientific Discovery of AIDS and the Quest for a Cure : Penguin, Harmondsworth.

Connor, S. and Kingman, S. 1989 The Search for the Virus : The Scientific Discovery of AIDS and the Quest for a Cure : Penguin, Harmondsworth.

Cooper, C.L. and Payne, R. (eds) 1978 Stress at Work : Wiley, Chichester.

Cooper, C.L. 1981 Stress Research : Wiley, Chichester.

Corey, F. 1983 I Never Knew I Had A Choice: 2nd Edition :Brooks-Cole, California.

Cormier, L.S.1987 The Professional Counsellor:a Process Guide to Helping Prentice Hall, Englewood Cliffs, New Jersey.

Corsini, R 1984 Current Psychotherapies : 3rd edition Peacock,Itasca, Illinois.

Cowles, K.V., Rodgers, B.L. 1991 When a Loved One Has AIDS : Care for the Significant Other : Journal of Psychosocial Nursing and Mental Health Services : 29 : 4 : 6 - 12.

Curran, J. and Monti, P. (eds) : Social Skills Training : A Practical Handbook for Assessment and Treatment : Guildford, New York.

Curtis, L., Sturm, G., Billing, D.R. and Anderson, J.D. 1989 At the Breaking Point : When Should An Overworked Nurse Bail Out? : Journal of Christian Nursing : 6 : 1 : 4 - 9.

D' Augeili, A.R. and Kennedy, S.P. 1989 An Evaluation of AIDS Prevention Brochures for University Women and Men : AIDS Education and Prevention : 1 : 2 : 134 - 140.

D'Augelli, A.R. 1989 AIDS Fears and Homophobia Among Rural Nursing Personnel : AIDS Education and Prevention : 1 : 4 : 277 - 284.

Daleo, R.E. 1986 Taking Care of the Caregivers : Five Strategies for Stamina : American Journal of Hospice Care : 3 : 5 : 33 - 38.

Daniels, V. and Horowitz, L.J. 1984 Being and Caring : A Psychology for Living : 2nd Edition : Mayfield, Mountain View, California.

Darling, L.W. 1986 What to do About Toxic Mentors : Nurse Educator : 11 : 2: 29 - 30.

Darling, L.A.W. 1984 What Do Nurses Want in a Mentor? : The Journal of Nursing Administration : October : 42 - 44.

Davidhizar, R., Boonstra, C., Lutz, K. and Poston, F. 1991 Teaching Safer Sex in Long Term Psychiatric Setting : Perspectives in Psychiatric Care : 27 : 1 : 25 - 29.

Davis, C.M. 1981 Affective Education for the Health Professions :Physical Therapy : 61 ; 11 : 1587 - 1593.

Dawley, H. and Wenrich, W. 1976 Achieving Assertive Behaviour : a Guide to Assertive Training : Brooks/Cole, Monterey, California.

De Vito, J.A. 1986 The Interpersonal Communication Book : 4th Edition : Harper and Row, New York.

Denker, A. 1989 Nursing Care of Children With Acquired Immunodeficiency Syndrome : A Grounded Theory Approach : University of Miami, Florida.

Dennis, H. 1991 AIDS : Getting the Message Nursing Times : 5 : 17 : 55 - 56.

Dickson, A. 1985 A Woman in Your Own Right : Assertiveness and You : Quartet Books, London.

Dilley, J.W., Pies, C. and Helquist, M. 1989 Face to Face : A Guide to AIDS Counseling : AIDS Health Project, University of California, San Francisco.

Dilley, J.W., Pies, C. and Helquist, M. 1989 Face to Face : a Guide to AIDS Counselling : AIDS Health Project, University of California, San Francisco, California.

Dixon, D.N. and Glover, J.A. 1984 Counselling : a problem solving approach : Wiley, Chichester.

Donoghue, M., Stimson, G. and Dolan, K. 1989 Sexual behaviour of injecting drug users and associated risks of HIV infection for non-injecting sexual partners : AIDS Care : 1 : 51 - 58.

Donoghue, M., Stimson, G. and Dolan, K. 1989 Sexual behaviour of injecting drug users and associated risks of HIV infection for non-injecting sexual partners : AIDS Care : 1 : 51 - 58.

Dowd, S.B. 1991 The Knowledge and Attitudes of Radiologic Technologists and Allied Health Students Regarding AIDS and AIDS Patients : Canadian Journal of Medical Radiation Technology : 22 : 1 : 19 - 22.

Dryden, W., Charles-Edwards and Woolfe, R. 1989 Handbook of Counselling in Britain : Routledge.

Du Bois, E.E. 1982 Human Resource Development : Expanding Role. In C. Klevens (ed) Materials and Methods in Adult and Continuing.

Duncan, S. and Fiske, D.W. 1977 Face - to - Face Interaction : Research, Methods and Theory : Lawrence Erlbaum Associates, Hillsdale, New Jersey.

Edelwich, J. Brondsky, A. 1980 Burnout : Stages of Disillusionment in the Helping Professions : Human Sciences Press, New York.

Eden, D. 1982 Critical Job Events, Acute Stress and Strain : Organisational Behaviour and Human Performance : 30 : 312 - 329.

Edmunds, M. 1983 The Nurse Preceptor Role :Nurse Practitioner : 8 : 6 : 52 - 53.

Edson, M. 1990 St Francis Central : One Organization Response to AIDS : Occupational Therapy in Health Care : 7 : 185 - 194.

Egan, G. 1986 Exercises in Helping Skills : 3rd edition :Brooks/Cole, Monterey, California.

Ellis R. and Whittington, D. 1981 A Guide to Social Skill Training : Croom Helm, London.

Ellis, R. and Whittington, D. (eds) 1983 : New Directions in Social Skills Training : Croom Helm, London.

Ellis, A. 1962 Reason and Emotion in Psychotherapy : Lyle, Stuart, New Jersey.

Ellis, R. (ed) 1989 Professional Competence and Quality Assurance in the Caring Professions : Chapman and Hall, London.

Epting, F. 1984 Personal Construct Counselling and Psychotherapy :Wiley, Chichester.

Ernst, S. and Goodison, L. 1981 In our Own Hands : a Book of Self Help Therapy :The Womens' Press, London.

Evans, D. (ed) 1990 Why Should We Care? : Macmillan, London.

Everly, G.S. and Rosenfeld, R. 1981 The Nature and Treatment of the Stress Response : a Practical Guide for Clinicians : Plenum Press, New York.

Fabry, J. 1968 The Pursuit of Meaning : Beacon Press, Boston, Mass.

Farber, B.A. (ed). 1983 Stress and Burnout in the Human Services : Pergamon Press, London.

Fay, A. 1978 Making Things Better By Making Them Worse : Hawthorne, New York.

Federal Centre for AIDS : 1987 Caring Together : The Report of the Expert Working Group on Integrated Palliative Care for Persons With AIDS : Federal Centre for AIDS, Health and Welfare, Canada.

Fedor, M.A. 1991 Advocacy and Activism : Nursing and Health Care : 12 : 3 : 119.

Feldenkrais, M.1972 Awareness Through Movement : Harper and Row, New York.

Fernando, S. 1990 Mental Health, Race and Culture : Macmillan, London.

Ferruci, P.1982 What We May Be :Turnstone Press, Wellingborough.

Field, P.A. and Morse, J.M. 1985 Nursing Research : The Application of Qualitative Approaches : Croom Helm, London.

Fielding, P. and Berman, P. (eds) 1989 Surviving in General Management : Macmillan, London.

Filley, A.C. 1975 Interpersonal Conflict Resolution : Scott, Foresman, Glenview, Illinois.

Fineman, S. 1985 Social Work Stress and Intervention : Gower, London.

Firth, J.A. 1986 Levels and Sources of Stress in Medical Students : British Medical Journal : 292 : 1177-1180.

Firth, J. 1985 Personal Meanings of Occupational Stress : Cases from the Clinic : Journal of Occupational Psychology : 58 : 139 - 148.

Firth, H., McKeown, P., McIntee, J. and Britton, P. 1987 Burn-Out, Personality and Support in Long-Stay Nursing :Nursing Times : 83 : 32 : 55 - 57.

Fisher, S. and Reason, J. 1988 Handbook of Life Stress : Cognition and Health : Wiley, Chichester.

Fisher, S. 1986 Stress and Strategy : Lawrence Erlbaum Associates, London.

Fitzpatrick, M. and Milligan, D. 1990 Reflections on the AIDS panic : Living Marxism : 15 : 14 - 19.

Fitzpatrick, M. and Milligan, D. 1990 Reflections on the AIDS panic : Living Marxism : 15 : 14 - 19.

Flaskerud, , J.H. 1987 AISA : Neuropsychiatric Complications Journal of Psychosocial Nursing and Mental Health Services : 25 : 17 - 20.

Foggo-Pays, E. 1983 An Introductory Guide to Counselling Ravenswood, Beckenham.

Fontana, D. 1989 Managing Stress : British Psychological Society and Routledge, London.

Fordham, F. 1966 An Introduction to Jung's Psychology : Penguin, Harmondsworth.

Fox, R.C., Aiken, L.H. and Messikomer, C.M. 1990 The Culture of Caring : AIDS and the Nursing Profession : Milbank Quarterly : 68 : 226 - 256.

France, R. and Robson, M. 1986, Behaviour Therapy in Primary Care.

Francis, D. and Young, D. 1979 Improving Work Groups : A Practical Manual for Team Building : University Associates, San Diego, California.

Frankenberg, R. 1990 Review article : Disease, literature and the body in the era of AIDS - a preliminary exploration : Sociology of Health and Illness : 12 : 3 : 351 - 359.

Frankenberg, R. 1990 Review article : Disease, literature and the body in the era of AIDS - a preliminary exploration : Sociology of Health and Illness : 12 : 3 : 351 - 359.

Frankl, V.E. 1959 Mans Search for Meaning : Beacon Press, New York.

Frankl, V.E. 1978 The Unheard Cry for Meaning : Simon and Schuster, New York.

Freemont, M. 1989 Memory Mate : Broderbund Software, San Rafael, California.

Freudenberger, H. and Richelson, G. 1974 Burnout : How to Beat the High Cost of Success : Bantam Books, New York.

Fromm, E. 1941 Escape from Freedom, Avon, New York.

Froner, G. and Rowniak, S. 1989 The Health Outreach Team : Taking AIDS Education and Health Care to the Streets : AIDS Education and Prevention : 1 : 2 : 105 - 118.

Fullilove, M.T. 1989 Ethnic Minorities, HIV disease and the growing underclass. In J.W. Dilley, C. Pies and M. Heliquist : Face to Face : A Guide to AIDS Counselling : AIDS Health Project, University of California, San Francisco, California.

Gallagher, R.M. and Cass, P.S. 1990 AIDS : Who Will Care at Home? AIDS Education and Prevention : 2 : 2 : 145 - 158.

Gallop, R., Taerk, G., Lancee, W., Coates, R., Fanning, M. and Keatings, M. 1991 Nurses and AIDS : Canadian Nurse : 87 : 1 : 29 - 31.

Gaze, H. 1987 Keep morals out : religious attitudes to AIDS : Nursing Times : 83 : 50 : 16 - 29.

Gaze, H. 1987 Keep morals out : religious attitudes to AIDS : Nursing Times : 83 : 50 : 16 - 29.

Gendlin, E.T. and Beebe, J. 1968 An Experiential Approach to Group Therapy :Journal of Research and Developments in Education: 1 : 19 - 29.

Gibson, R.L. and Mitchell, M.H.1986 Introduction to Counselling and Guidance Collier Macmillan, London.

Goffman, I. 1971 The Presentation of Self in Everyday Life : Penguin, Harmondsworth.

Goldberg, L and Beznitz, S. 1982 Handbook of Stress : Theoretical and Clinical Aspects : Macmillan, New York.

Green, J. and Miller, D. 1986 AIDS : The Story of a Disease : Grafton Books, London.

H.M.S.O. 1987 AIDS : Monitoring Response to the Public Education Campaign : February 1986 - February 1987 : HMSO, London.

Halmos, P. 1965 The Faith of the Counsellors : Constable, London.

Hancock, C. 1991 AIDS : The Challenge for Nurses : Nursing Standard : 16 : 5 : 50 - 52.

Hancock, C. 1991 AIDS Focus : The Challenge for Nurses : Nursing Standard : 5 : 17 : 50 - 52.

Hancock, C. 1991 AIDS Focus : The Challenge for Nurses : Nursing Standard : 5 : 17 : 50 - 52.

Hargie, O., Saunders, C. and Dickson, D. 1981 Social Skills in Interpersonal Communication : 2nd Edition : Croom Helm, London.

Hargie, O., Saunders, C. and Dickson, D. 1981 Social Skills in Interpersonal Communication : 2nd Edition :Croom Helm, London.

Hargie, O. (ed) 1987 A Handbook of Communication Skills : Croom Helm, London.

Harris, T.1969 I'm O.K., Your O.K. : Harper and Row, London.

Harvey, N. 1991 The Psychosocial Context of AIDS/HIV : Nursing Standard : 5 : 27 : 50 - 51.

Hawkins, P. and Shohet, R. 1989 Supervision and the Helping Professions :Open University Press, Milton Keynes.

Health Education Authority : High Stress Occupation Working Party : 1988 : Stress in the Public Sector : Nurses, Police, Social Workers and Teachers : Health Education Authority.

Hegarty, M.C. 1990 Psychological and Social Consequences...AIDS : World Health : Nov-Dec : 18 - 19.

Heginbotham, C. 1990 Mental Health, Human Rights and Legislation : Macmillan, London.

Heins, M., Fahey, S.N. and Leiden, L.I. 1984 Perceived Stress in Medical, Law and Graduate Students : Journal of Medical Education : 59 : 169 - 179.

Herinck, R. (ed)1980 The Psychotherapy Handbook New American Library, New York.

Heron , J. 1978 Co-Counselling Teachers Manual : Human Potential Research Project, University of Surrey, Guildford.

Heron, J. 1990 Helping the Client : Sage, London.

Heron, J. 1977 Behaviour Analysis in Education and Training : Human Potential Research Project : University of Surrey, Guildford, Surrey.

Heron, J. 1973 Experiential Training Techniques :Human Potential Research Project, University of Surrey, Guildford.

Heron, J. 1980 Paradigm Papers :Human Potential Research Project, University of Surrey, Guildford.

Heron, J. 1977 Catharsis in Human Development : Human Potential Research Project : University of Surrey, Guildford, Surrey.

Heron, J. 1977 Behaviour Analysis in Education and Training :Human Potential Research Project, University of Surrey,Guildford.

Howard, G.S., Nance, D.W. and Meyers, P. 1987 Adaptive Counselling and Therapy:a systematic approach to selecting effective treatments :Jossey bass, San Francisco, California.

Howe, J. 1989 AIDS - The rights approach : Professional Nurse : 5 : 3 : 156 - 159.

Hughes, J. 1987 Cancer and Emotion : Wiley, Chichester.

Hull, D. and Schroeder, H. 1979 Some Interpersonal Effects of Assertion, Non-Assertion and Aggression :Behaviour Therapy : 10: 20 - 29.

Hurding, R.F.1985 Roots and Shoots : a guide to counselling and psychotherapy Hodder and Stoughton, London.

Hurtig, W. and Fandrick, C. 1990 The nursing student and the psychiatric patient with AIDS : a case study : Nurse Education Today : 10 : 2 : 92 - 97.

Hutchins, D.E.1987 Helping Relationships and Strategies Brooks-Cole, Monterey, California.

Ivey, A.E.1987 Counselling and Psychotherapy : Skills, theories and practice : Prentice Hall International, London.

Jacobson, D. 1989 Context and the Sociological Study of Stress : an Invited Response to Pearlin : Journal of Health and Social Behaviour : 30 : 3 : 257 - 260.

Johnson, D.W. and Johnson, F.P. 1982 Joining Together : 2nd Edition : Prentice Hall, Englewood Cliffs, New Jersey.

Johnson, D.W. 1972 Reaching Out : Prentice Hall, Englewood Cliffs, New Jersey.

Johnson, A. and Gill, O. 1989 Evidence for recent changes in the sexual behaviour of homosexual men. Phil. Trans. R. Soc. Lond. : B325 : 153 - 61.

Jones, J.G., Janman, K., Payne, R.L. and Rick, J.T. 1987 Some Determinants of Stress in Psychiatric Nurses : International Journal of Nursing Studies : 24 : 2 : 129 - 144.

Jourard, S. 1964 The Transparent Self : Van Nostrand, Princeton, New Jersey.

Jourard, S. 1971 Self-Disclosure : an Experimental Analysis of the Transparent Self : Wiley, New York.

Jung, C.G. 1976 Modern Man in Search of a Soul :Routledge and Kegan Paul, London.

Kelly, C. 1979 Assertion Training : A Facilitator's Guide : University Associates : La Jolla, California.

Kelly, C. 1979 Assertion Training : A Facilitator's Guide : University Associates La Jolla, California.

Kennedy, E. 1979 On Becoming a Counsellor Gill and Macmillan, London.

Kilpatrick, W. 1988 AIDS : Sharing the Pain : Pastoral Guidelines :Darton, Longman and Todd, London.

Kilty, J. 1978 Self and Peer Assessment:Human Potential Research Project.

Kilty, J. 1987 Staff Development for Nurse Education :Practitioners Supporting Students : A Report of a 5-Day Development Workshop :Human Potential Research Project : University of Surrey, Guildford.

King, E.C. 1984 Affective Education in Nursing : A Guide to Teaching and Assessment :Aspen, Maryland.

Kirkpatrick, W. 1988 AIDS : Sharing the Pain : Pastoral Guidelines : Darton, Longman and Todd, London.

Kitzinger, J. 1990 Audience understandings of AIDS media messages : a discussion of methods : Sociology of Health And

Illness : 12 : 3 : 319 - 335.

Kitzinger, J. 1990 Audience understandings of AIDS media messages : a discussion of methods : Sociology of Health And Illness : 12 : 3 : 319 - 335.

Kizer, W.M. 1987 The Health Workplace : A Blueprint for Corporate Action : Delmar, London.

Klimes, I, Catalan, J., Bond, A. and Day, A. 1989 Knowledge and Attitudes of Health Care Staff About HIV Infection in a Health Care District With Low HIV Prevalence : 1 : 3 : 313 - 317.

Knox, M.D. , Dow, M.G. and Cotton, D.A. 1989 Mental Health Care Providers : the Need for AIDS Education : AIDS Education and Prevention : 1 : 4 : 285 - 290.

Kopp, S.1974 If You Meet the Buddha on the Road, Kill Him! :A Modern Pilgrimage Through Myth, Legend and Psychotherapy : Sheldon Press, London.

Kottler, J.A. and Brown, R.W. 1985 Introduction to Therapeutic Counselling Brooks-Cole, Monterey, California.

L' Abate, L. and Milan, M. (eds) 1985 Handbook of Social Skills Training and Research : Wiley, New York.

Lachman, V.D. 1983 Stress Management : a Manual for Nurses : Grune and Stratton, Orlando, Florida.

Lang, A.J. and Jakubowski, P. 1978 The Assertive Option : Research Press, Champagne.

Langone, J. 1988 AIDS : The Facts : Little Brown, Boston.

Larson, D.G. 1986 Developing Effective Hospice Staff Support Groups : Pilot Test of an Innovative Training Programs : Hospice Journal : 2 : 2 : 41 - 55.

Last, J.M. 1988 Natural and Social History of Epidemics : AIDS : A Perspective for Canadians : Background Papers : Royal

Society of Canada, Ontario.

Last, J.M. 1988 Natural and Social History of Epidemics : AIDS : A Perspective for Canadians : Background Papers : Royal Society of Canada, Ontario.

Lazarus, R.S. and Folkman, S. 1984 Stress, Appraising and Coping : Springer, New York.

Leech, K. 1986 Spirituality and Pastoral Care : Sheldon Press, London.

Leukefeld, C.G. 1988 AIDS counselling and testing : Health and Social Work : 13 : 3 : 167 - 169.

Lovejoy, N.C. and Moran, T.A. 1988 Selected AIDS beliefs, behaviours and informational needs of homosexual/bisexual men with AIDS or ARC : International Journal of Nursing Studies : 25 : 3 : 207 - 216.

MacCaffrey, E.A. 1987 Counselling AIDS patients : a unique approach by Shanti therapists : AIDS Patient Care : 1 : 2 : 26 - 27.

Marshall, E.K. and Kurtz, P.D. (eds) 1982 Interpersonal Helping Skills : A guide to Training Methods, Programs and Resources : Jossey Bass, San Francisco, California.

Marshall, T.A. and Nieckarz, J.P. 1988 Bereavement Counselling : AIDS Patient Care : 2 : 2 : 21 - 25.

Marzuk, P., Tierney, J., Tardiff, K., Gross, E.M., Morgan, E.B. and Hsu, M.A. et al 1988 Increased risk of suicide in persons with AIDS Journal of the American Medical Association : 259 : 1333-1337.

McGough, K.N. 1990 Assessing social support for people with AIDS : Oncology Nursing Forum : 17 : 1 : 31 - 35.

McNicol, L.B., Hadersbeck, R.E., Dickens, D.R. and Brown, J.E. 1991 AIDS and Pregnancy : Survey of Knowledge, Attitudes, Beliefs and Self-Identification of Risk : Journal of Obstetrics, Gynaecological and Neonatal Nursing : 20 : 1 : 65 - 72.

Mayeroff, M. 1972 On Caring : Harper and Row, New York.

Miller, C. 1990 The AIDS Handbook : Penguin, Harmondsworth.

Miller, D., Weber, J. and Green, J. (eds) 1986 The Management of AIDS Patients : Macmillan, London.

Miller, D. 1987 Living With AIDS and HIV : Macmillan, London.

Miller, C. 1990 The AIDS Handbook : Penguin, Harmondsworth.

Moreno, J.L. 1969 Psychodrama Vol III : Beacon House Press, Beacon, New York.

Moreno, J.L. 1959 Psychodrama Vol II : Beacon House Press, Beacon, New York.

Moreno, J.L. 1977 Psychodrama, Vol I : 4th Edition: Beacon House Press, Beacon, New York.

Morley, I.E. 1987 Negotiating and Bargaining. In Hargie, O. (ed) A Handbook of Communication Skills : Croom Helm, London.

Morley, I.E. 1982 Preparation for Negotiating L Conflict, Commitment and Choice. In Bradstatter, H., Davis, J.H. and Stocker - Kreichgauer, G. (eds) Group Decision Making : Academic Press, London.

Morrison, P., Burnard, P. and Hackett, P. 1991 A Smallest Space Analysis of Nurses' Perceptions of Their Interpersonal Skills : Counselling Psychology Quarterly : 4 : 2/3 : 119 - 125.

Morrison, P. and Burnard, P. 1991 Student's Views on Counselling : Journal of District Nursing : 10 : 2 : 11 - 13.

Morrison, P. and Burnard, P. 1989 Students' and Trained Nurses' Perceptions of Their Own Interpersonal Skills : a report and comparison : Journal of Advanced Nursing : 14 : 321 - 329.

Morrison, P. and Burnard, P. 1990 Interpersonal Skills : A Smallest Space Analysis : Nursing Times : 86 : 14 : 55.

Morrison, P. and Burnard, P. 1988 Clarifying Nurses' Interpersonal Skills : Nursing Times : 84 : 30 : 49.

Morrison, P., Burnard, P. and Hackett, P. (1991) A smallest space analysis of nurses' perceptions of their interpersonal skills. Counselling Psychology Quarterly, 4, 2/3, 115-121.

Morrison, P. (1988) Nurses' perceptions of caring. Nursing Times, 84, 9, 51.

Morrison, P. and Burnard, P. (1990) Interpersonal skills: a smallest space analysis. Nursing Times, 86, 14, 55.

Morrison, P. (1990) An example of the use of repertory grid technique in assessing nurse's self-perceptions of caring. Nurse Education Today, 10, 253-259.

Morrison, P. (1989) The caring attitude : nurses' self-perceptions. Nursing Times, 85, 4, 56.

Morrison, P. (1990) A multidimensional scalogram analysis of the use of seclusion in acute psychiatric settings. Journal of Advanced Nursing, 15, 59-66.

Morsund, J.1985 The Process of Counselling and Therapy Prentice Hall, Englewood Cliffs, New Jersey.

Munro, A., Manthei, B. and Small, J.1988 Counselling : The Skills of Problem-Solving :Routledge, London.

Murgatroyd, S. and Woolfe, R. 1982 Coping with Crisis-Understanding and Helping Persons in Need : Harper and Row,London.

Murgatroyd, S. 1986 Counselling and Helping :British Psychological Society and Methuen, London.

Neighbors, M. and Henderson, M. 1991 What Nurses Don't Know About AIDS : Advancing Clinical Care : 6 : 2 : 27.

Nelkin, D. 1987 AIDS and the social sciences : review of

useful knowledge and research needs : Review of Infectious Diseases : 9 : 947 - 60.

Nelson-Jones, R. 1984 Personal Responsibility: counselling and therapy : an integrative approach : Harper and Row, London.

Nelson-Jones, R. 1988 Practical Counselling and Helping Skills: helping clients to help themselves :Cassell, London.

Nelson-Jones, R.1983 Practical Counselling Skills : a psychological skills approach for the helping professions and for voluntary counsellors Holt Rinehart and Winston, London.

Nelson-Jones, R. 1981 The Theory and Practice of Counselling Psychology :Holt Rinehart and Winston, London.

Nichols, S.E., Ostrow, D.G. : Psychiatric Implication of Acquired Immune Deficiency Syndrome : American Psychiatric Press, Washington.

Okoneski, D. 1990 Gay Grief : Issues of Love, Loss and Loneliness : Occupational Therapy in Health Care : 7 : 213 - 226.

Open University Coping With Crisis Group 1987 Running Workshops : A Guide for Trainers in the Helping Professions :Croom Helm, London.

Osborn, S.M. and Harris, G.G. 1975 Assertive Training for Women : Charles C. Thomas, Springfield, Illinois.

Palmer, M.E. and Deck, E.S. 1982 Assertiveness Education : One Method for Teaching Staff and Patients : Nurse Educator : Winter : 36 - 39.

Payne, R. and Firth-Conzens, J. (eds) 1987 Stress in Health Professionals : Wiley, Chichester.

Perry, E. and Tross, S. 1984 Psychiatric problems of AIDS inpatients at the New York Hospital Public Health Representative : 99 : 200 - 205.

Perry, S. and Tross, S. 1984 Psychiatric problems of AIDS inpatients at the New York Hospital : a Preliminary Report : Public Health Reports : 99 : 200 - 205.

Polk-Walker, G.C. 1989 Treatment of AIDS in a psychiatric setting Perspectives in Psychiatric Care : XXV ; 2 : 9 - 13.

Pommerance, L.M. and Shields, J.J. 1989 Factors Associated With Hospital Workers' Reactions to the Treatment of Persons With AIDS : Aids Education and Prevention : 1 : 3 : 184 - 193.

Pratt, R.J. 1988 AIDS : A Strategy for Nursing Care : Arnold, London.

Procter, B 1978 Counselling Shop: an Introduction to the theories and techniques of ten approaches to counselling Deutsch, London.

Pye, M., Kapila, M., Buckley, G. and Cunningham, D. (eds). 1989 Local AIDS Programmes in the UK : Longman, London.

Pye, M., Kapila, M., Buckley, G. and Cunningham, D. (eds). 1989 Local AIDS Programmes in the UK : Longman, London.

Rankin-Box, D.F. 1987 Complementary Health Therapies : A Guide for Nurses and the Caring Professions : Chapman and Hall, London.

Rawlings, M.E. and Rawlings, L. 1983 Mentoring and Networking for Helping Professionals : Personnel and Guidance Journal :62 : 2 : 116 -118.

Read, V. 1990 HIV/AIDS : Coping With The Stressors : Australian Nurses Journal : 20 : 5 : 15 - 16.

Read, V. 1990 Women and AIDS : Australian Nurses Journal : 20 : 4 : 22 - 24.

Reddy, M. 1987 The Manager's Guide to Counselling at Work Methuen, London.

Roffman, R.A. et al 1990 Continuing unsafe sex : assessing the need for AIDS prevention counselling : Public Health Reports :

105 : 2 : 202 - 208.

Rogers, C.R. and Stevens, B. 1967 Person to Person : The Problem of Being Human :Real People Press, Lafayette, California.

Rogers, C.R. 1951 Client-Centred Therapy : Constable, London.

Rogers, C.R. 1983 Freedom to Learn for the Eighties : Merrill, Columbus, Ohio.

Rogers, C.R. 1967 On Becoming a Person : Constable, London.
Rogers, C.R. 1985 Toward a More Human Science of the Person : Journal of Humanistic Psychology : 25 : 4 : 7-24.

Rothenberger, J.H. and Hochhauser, M. 1990 Chemical Dependency Counselor Attitudes and Opinions on AIDS : Addictions Nursing Network : 2 : 2 : 19 - 22.

Rotheram - Borus, M.J. and Koopman, C. 1991 Sexual Risk Behaviours, AIDS Knowledge and Beliefs About AIDS Among Runaways : American Journal of Public Health : 81 : 2 : 208 - 210.

Rowan, J.1986 Holistic Listening :Journal of Humanistic Psychology : 26 : 1 : 83 - 102.

Schulman, D. 1982 Intervention in Human Services : A guide to skills and knowledge : 3rd Edition : C.V. Mosby : St Louis, Missouri.

Scott, W.P. 1981 The Skills of Negotiating : Gower, Aldershot.

Scott, W.P. 1986 The Skills of Communicating : Gower, Aldershot.

Shafer, P. 1978 Humanistic Psychology :Prentice Hall,Englewood Cliffs, New Jersey.

Shafer, P. 1978 Humanistic Psychology : Prentice Hall,Englewood Cliffs, New Jersey.

Shamian, J. and Inhaber, R. 1985 The Concept and Practice of Preceptorship in Contemporary Nursing : A Review of Pertinent Literature : The International Journal of Nursing Studies : 22 : 2 : 79 - 88.

Shapiro, E.C., Haseltime, F, and Rowe, M. 1978 Moving Up : Role Models, Mentors and The Patron System : Sloan Management Review : 19 : 51 - 58.

Shaw, M.E. 1981 : Group Dynamics : The Psychology of Small Group Behaviour : McGraw Hill, New York.

Shostak, A.B. 1980 Blue-Collar Stress : Addison-Wesley, Reading, Masss.

Silven, D. and Caldarola, T.J. 1989 The HIV-Positive Client. In J.W. Dilley, C. Pies and M. Helquist : Face to Face : A Guide to AIDS Counselling : AIDS Health Project, University of California, San Francisco, California.

Silverman, D. and Perakyla, A. 1990 AIDS counselling : the interactional organisation of talk about 'delicate' issues : Sociology of Health and Illness : 12 : 3 : 293 - 317.

Sketchley, J. 1989 Counselling people affected by HIV and AIDS. In W. Dryden, D.Charles-Edwards and R. Woolfe : Handbook of Counselling in Britain. Tavistock/Routledge.

Sliverman, D. and Perakyla, A. 1990 AIDS counselling : the interactional organisation of talk about 'delicate' issues : Sociology of Health and Illness : 12 : 3 : 293 - 317.

Sontag, S. 1988 Aids and its metaphors : Allen Lane, Harmondsworth.

Sorensen, A.A. 1991 AIDS : What Should We Do : Pennyslvania Nurse : 46 : 1 : 9 - 11.

Spiegel, L. and Mayers, A. 1991 Psychosocial Aspects of AIDS in Children and Adolescents : Pediatric Clinics of North America : 38 : 1 : 153 - 167.

Strang, J. and Stimpson, G. (eds) 1990 AIDS and Drug Misuse : Routledge, London.

Strunin, L. 1991 Adolescents' Perceptions of Risk for HIV Infection : Social Science and Medicine : 32 : 2 : 221 - 228.

Sultan, G. 1991 How Much is Known About HIV? Nursing : 4 : 28 : 14 - 17.

Swanson, B., Cronin-Stubbs, Colleti, M.A. 1990 Dementia and depression in persons with AIDS : Causes and Care Journal of Psychosocial Nursing : 28 : 10 : 33 - 38.

Taylor, E. 1988 Anger Intervention : American Journal of Occupational Therapy : 42 : 3 : 147 - 155.

Thomas, B.1990 AIDS Research : The Human Side Nursing Times : 86 : 28 : 28 - 30.

Trower, P., Bryant, B.M. and Argyle, M. (eds) : Social Skills and Mental Health : Methuen, London.

Truax, C.B. and Carkuff, R.R. 1967 Towards Effective Counselling and Psychotherapy : Aldine, Chicago.

Tschudin, V. 1986 Counselling Skills for Nurses :Balliere Tindall, London.

Tschudin, V. 1991 Counselling Skills for Nurses : 3rd Edition : Balliere Tindall, London.

Tshudin, V. and Schober, J. 1990 Managing Yourself : Macmillan, London.

Walker, R. (ed) 1985 Applied Qualitative Research : Gower, Aldershot.

Wallace, W.A. 1986 Theories of Counselling and Psychotherapy : a basic issues approach Allyn and Bacon, Boston.

Wallis, R. 1984 Elementary Forms of the New Religious

Life : Routledge and Kegan Paul, London.

Warner-Robbins, C.G. and Christiana, N.M. 1989 The spiritual needs of persons with AIDS : Family and Community Health : 12 : 2 : 43 - 51.

Wass, H., Miller, M.D. and Thornton, G. 1990 AIDS Education in the US Public Schools : AIDS Education and Prevention : 2 : 3 : 213 - 219.

Watkins, J. 1978 The Therapeutic Self :Human Science Press, New York.

Welch, J. and Newbury, J. 1990 Looking After People with Late HIV Disease The Patten Press in association with the Lisa Sainsbury Foundation.

Wellings, K. and Wadsworth, J. 1990 AIDS and the moral Climate. In Jowell, R, Witherspoon, S. and Brooks, L. (eds) British Social Attitudes : the 7th Report : Gower, Aldershot.

Willis, D.J. 1990 A Survey of Nurses Attitudes To AIDS Related Issues : New Zealand Nursing Forum : 18 : 4 : 7 - 9.

Wilson, D., Wilson, C., Greenspan, R., Sibanda, P. and Msimanga, S. 1989 Towards an AIDS Strategy for Zimabwe : AIDS Education and Prevention : 1 : 2 : 96 - 104.

Wood, W. and Aull, M.R. 1990 Women and AIDS : Implications for Occupational Therapists : Occupational Therapy in Health Care : 7 : 151 - 160.

Wyatt, H.V. 1989 Ambiguities and Scares in Educational Material About AIDS : AIDS Education and Prevention : 1 : 2 : 119 - 125.

Yelin, E.H., Greenblatt, R.M., Hoolander, H. and McMaster, J.R. 1991 The Impact of HIV Related Illness on Employment : American Journal of Public Health : 81 : 1 : 79 - 84.

Index